GENERAL PR

The Clinical Survival Guide

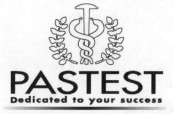

PASTEST
Dedicated to your success

Dedication

This book is dedicated to my husband Alistair and to my parents. Thank you for all your support over the past few months.

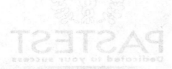

GENERAL PRACTICE
The Clinical Survival Guide

Rupal Shah

MBBS (Hons) MRCGP DRCOG

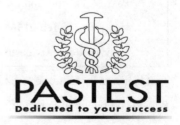

PASTEST
Dedicated to your success

© 2005 PASTEST Ltd

Egerton Court
Parkgate Estate
Knutsford
Cheshire
WA16 8DX

Telephone: 01565 752000

First published 2005

ISBN: 1 904627 44 7

A catalogue record for this book is available from the British Library.

The information contained within this book was obtained by the authors from reliable sources. However, while every effort has been made to ensure its accuracy, no responsibility for loss, damage or injury occasioned to any person acting or refraining from action as a result of information contained herein can be accepted by the publishers or authors.

Every effort has been made to contact holders of copyright to obtain permission to reproduce copyright material. However, if any have been inadvertently overlooked, the publisher will be pleased to make the necessary arrangements at the first opportunity.

Text prepared by Carnegie Book Production, Lancaster

Printed and bound in Europe by the Alden Group

Contents

Foreword

When I first started as a general practitioner (GP), I found myself regularly bewildered by the number of startlingly obscure questions I was asked by patients, most of which didn't seem to have been covered in any way by my medical training. The idea for this book was born from these experiences and its aim is to go some way towards filling in the gaps of knowledge left after completing medical school, house jobs and most standard vocational training schemes. It comprises subjects that I did not feel fully equipped to deal with when I started my registrar year. It is therefore by no means a comprehensive medical textbook, but is meant as a guide, providing practical advice on some of the more obscure topics which GPs are often faced with, as well as up-to-date guidelines on the management of common conditions.

Acknowledgements

The Orthopaedics chapter was written by Mr Alistair Tindall, MBBS MRCS(Eng), Specialist Registrar, South East Thames rotation.

The ENT chapter was written by Mr Alex Bennett, MBBS MRCS DLO, Specialist Registrar, Eastern Deanery.

The Urology chapter was written by Mr Peter Acher MA MRCS, Mr Tony Young FRCS, Specialist Registrar, South East Thames rotation.

Many thanks to the following for their help and advice in writing this book:

- Dr Ashley Conway   Consultant Psychotherapist, New Cavendish Street Surgery, London

- Dr David Westaby   Consultant Gastroenterologist, Chelsea and Westminster Hospital, London

- Dr Nick Wales   Consultant Gynaecologist, Chelsea and Westminster Hospital, London

- Dr Richard Morgan   Consultant Physician, Chelsea and Westminster Hospital, London

- Dr Kevin Fox   Consultant Cardiologist, Charing Cross Hospital, London

- Dr Christine Costello   Consultant Haematologist, Chelsea and Westminster Hospital, London

- Dr Karim Meeran   Consultant Endocrinologist, Chelsea and Westminster Hospital, London

- Dr Christopher Bridgett   Consultant Psychiatrist, Chelsea and Westminster Hospital, London

- Dr Michael Feher   Consultant Endocrinologist, Chelsea and Westminster Hospital, London

- Dr Paul Holloway   Consultant Biochemist, St Mary's Hospital, London

- Dr Chaulanie de Silva   SpR Rheumatology, St George's Hospital, London

- Dr Miriam Antoniou   MCSP Community paediatric physiotherapist, London

Glossary

AA	Alcoholics Anonymous
ACBS	Advisory Committee on Borderline Substances
ACE	Angiotensin-converting enzyme
ACL	Anterior cruciate ligament
ACR	American College of Rheumatology
AD	Alzheimer's disease
AFP	Alpha-fetoprotein
ALOs	*Actinomyces*-like organisms
ALP	Alkaline phosphatase
ALT	Alanine aminotransferase
AMD	Acute macular degeneration
AML	Acute myelogenous leukaemia
ANA	Antinuclear antibody
ANCA	Anti-neutrophil cytoplasm autoantibodies
anti-TPO	Antithyroid peroxidase
ARBs	Angiotensin-receptor blockers
AST	Aspartate transaminase
ASW	Approved social worker
AUDIT	Alcohol Use Disorders Identification Test
AVN	Avascular necrosis
BAHA	Bone-anchored hearing aids
BHS	British Hypertension Society
BMD	Bone mineral density
BNP	B-type natriuretic peptide
BXO	Balanitis xerotica obliterans
CABG	Coronary artery bypass graft
CBT	Cognitive behavioural therapy
CHD	Coronary heart disease
CIN	Cervical intraepithelial neoplasia
CMPA	Cow's milk protein allergy
CMV	Cytomegalovirus
CNS	Central nervous system
COCP	Combined oral contraceptive pill
COPD	Chronic obstructive pulmonary disease
COX-2	Cyclooxygenase-2
CRP	C-reactive protein
CSM	Committee on Safety of Medicines
CVA	Cerebrovascular accident
CVD	Cardiovascular disease
CXR	Chest X-ray

D&C	Dilation and curettage
DEXA	Dual-energy X-ray absorptiometry
DIC	Disseminated intravascular coagulation
DLA	Disability Living Allowance
DMARDs	Disease-modifying antirheumatic drugs
DoH	Department of Health
DRE	Digital rectal examination
dsDNA	Double-stranded DNA
DVLA	Driver and Vehicle Licensing Agency
DVT	Deep vein thrombosis
EBV	Epstein–Barr virus
ED	Erectile dysfunction
EPDS	Edinburgh Postnatal Depression Scale
ENA	Extractable nuclear antigen
EPSEs	Extrapyramidal side-effects
ERIC	Enuresis Resource and Information Centre
ESR	Erythrocyte sedimentation rate
FBC	Full blood count
FVS	Fetal varicella syndrome
GBS	Group B *Streptococcus*
GDS	Geriatric Depression Scale
GGT	Gamma-glutamyl transferase
GI	Gastrointestinal
GMS	General Medical Services
GnRH	Gonadotrophin-releasing hormone
GP	General practitioner
H_2RA	H_2-receptor antagonist
Hb	Haemoglobin
hCG	Human chorionic gonadotrophin
HDL	High-density lipoprotein
HPV	Human papillomavirus
HRT	Hormone replacement therapy
IBS	Irritable bowel syndrome
IMB	Intermenstrual bleeding
IPSS	International Prostate Symptom Score
ISMN	Isosorbide mononitrate
ITP	Idiopathic (autoimmune) thrombocytopenia
IUD	Intrauterine device
LFTs	Liver function tests
LH	Luteinising hormone
LUTS	Lower urinary tract symptoms
LVD	Left ventricular dysfunction
LVH	Left ventricular hypertrophy

MCI	Mild cognitive impairment
MCP	Metacarpophalangeal
MCPJs	Metacarpophalangeal joints
MCV	Mean cell volume
MGUS	Monoclonal gammopathy of unknown significance
MI	Myocardial infarction
MLD	Manual lymphatic drainage
MMSE	Mini mental state examination
MRI	Magnetic resonance imaging
MSU	Mid-stream urine
MTP	Metatarsophalangeal
NASH	Non-alcoholic steatohepatitis
NICE	National Institute for Clinical Excellence
NSAIDs	Non-steroidal anti-inflammatory drugs
OA	Osteoarthritis
OE	Otitis externa
OTC	Over the counter
PAD	Peripheral artery disease
PAPP-A	Pregnancy-associated plasma protein A
PCOS	Polycystic ovarian syndrome
PCR	Polymerase chain reaction
PCV	Packed cell volume
PD	Parkinson's disease
PDE	Phosphodiesterase
PID	Pelvic inflammatory disease
PIP	Proximal interphalangeal
PMR	Polymyalgia rheumatica
PMS	Premenstrual syndrome
POP	Progesterone-only pill
PPI	Proton pump inhibitor
PSA	Prostate-specific antigen
PUD	Peptic ulcer disease
PUJ	Pelvi-ureteric junction
RA	Rheumatoid arthritis
RAST	Radioallergosorbent
RR	Relative risk
SHBG	Sex hormone-binding globulin
SIADH	Syndrome of inappropriate antidiuretic hormone (secretion)
SIGN	Scottish Intercollegiate Guidelines Network
SLE	Systemic lupus erythematosus
SMP	Statutory Maternity Pay
SNRIs	Serotonin and noradrenaline reuptake inhibitors
SSRIs	Selective serotonin reuptake inhibitors

STDs	Sexually transmitted diseases
SUFE	Slipped upper femoral epiphysis
SX	Symptom
TB	Tuberculosis
TCAs	Tricyclic antidepressants
TFTs	Thyroid function tests
TIA	Transient ischaemic attack
TMJ	Temporomandibular joint
TSH	Thyroid-stimulating hormone
TTG	Tissue transglutaminase
TURP	Transurethral resection of the prostate
TVT	Tension-free vaginal taping
TZDs	Thiazolidinediones
UC	Ulcerative colitis
U&Es	Urea and electrolytes
UTI	Urinary tract infection
VTE	Venous thromboembolism
VZIG	Varicella zoster immunoglobulin
WHO	World Health Organisation

CHAPTER 1
CARDIOVASCULAR DISEASE

CHAPTER 1
CARDIOVASCULAR DISEASE

CHAPTER 1
CARDIOVASCULAR DISEASE

For this chapter, it is worth noting that coronary heart disease (CHD) refers to myocardial infarction (MI), angina and coronary artery disease (eg patients who have had bypass operations or angioplasties).

The term 'cardiovascular disease' (CVD) incorporates cerebrovascular disease and peripheral vascular disease, as well as CHD. The CVD risk can be calculated by multiplying the CHD risk by 4/3: for example, a CHD risk of 15% is equivalent to a CVD risk of 20%. CVD risk is a more important measurement than CHD risk in many ways and has been used in the latest Joint British Society risk charts.

Treatment guidelines are becoming ever more stringent, with drugs for primary prevention being started earlier and earlier; there seems to be a danger that if this trend continues, most of the older UK population will end up on medication to prevent CVD. However, it should never be forgotten that most CVD can be prevented by modifying lifestyle factors: for example, smoking 6–10 cigarettes a day doubles the risk of MI, while smoking 20 cigarettes increases the risk fourfold and smoking 40 cigarettes leads to a ninefold increase in risk.

HYPERTENSION

The British Hypertension Society (BHS) updated their guidance in 2004, based on evidence from several large-scale studies. These guidelines have proved to be quite controversial and many GPs feel that the targets are unrealistic and too complicated, especially in their cholesterol recommendations. A more pragmatic approach is to reduce blood pressure to the lowest level that the patient can tolerate.

The BHS classification of hypertension is summarised in Table 1.1:

	Blood pressure (mmHg)	
	Systolic	Diastolic
Optimal BP	<120	<80
Normal BP	<130	<85
High – normal BP	130–139	85–89
Grade 1 hypertension	140–159	90–99
Grade 2 hypertension	160–179	100–109
Grade 3 hypertension	>180	>110
Isolated systolic hypertension (grade 1)	140–159	<90
Isolated systolic hypertension (grade 2)	>160	<90

Table 1.1: BHS classification of hypertension (with copyright permission from the British Hypertension Society, 'BHS classification of blood pressure levels,' *Journal of Human Hypertension*, 2004, 18, p.142, Box 1)

In the USA, patients with high–normal BPs are labelled as having 'pre-hypertension'. Fortunately, given the huge number of people who would fall into this 'disease category', the term is not yet being used in the UK!

MONITORING BP (ACCORDING TO THE BHS)

- All adults should routinely have their BP monitored every 5 years.

- Adults with high–normal BPs and those who have had high readings at any time in the past should have their BP measured annually (if implemented, this would mean a hugely increased workload for GPs, particularly in terms of monitoring patients with 'high–normal' BPs).

- An appropriate size of cuff should be used, such that the bladder covers at least 80% of the upper arm. Using a cuff that is too small will lead to an overestimation of BP and vice versa. There are three sizes of cuff available.

- The BP should be measured with the arm supported at heart level.

NOTE: Elderly patients often have a postural drop in BP. Therefore, in these patients, BP should also be measured when they are standing (after at least 2 minutes standing). If there is a postural drop of >20 mmHg, use the standing BP.

ESTABLISHING THE DIAGNOSIS

BP is very variable, particularly in the elderly. It is therefore recommended to measure BP on a minimum of three different occasions (but ideally more) before initiating therapy. Treatment may be needed if **either** the systolic BP **or** the diastolic BP is raised.

- For grade 1 hypertensives (**BP 140–159/90–99 mmHg**) without diabetes, target organ damage (eg left ventricular hypertrophy (LVH) or renal impairment) or cardiovascular disease (CVD), confirm the diagnosis by taking two measurements per visit, repeated monthly over 4–6 months. Decide on whether to treat according to CVD risk (treat if >20% over 10 years).

- For grade 1 hypertensives with diabetes, target organ damage or CVD, confirm the diagnosis of hypertension over the course of 3 months, and then treat.

- For grade 2 hypertensives (**BP 160–179/100–109 mmHg**), confirm the diagnosis over 1–3 months and start treatment. For grade 2 hypertensive patients with complications, confirm over 3–4 weeks, and then treat; everybody with a BP of >160/100 mmHg needs treatment.

- For grade 3 hypertensives (**BP >180/110 mmHg**), confirm over 1–2 weeks, and then treat. Immediate treatment is needed if the BP is >220/120 mmHg; this should be according to normal treatment guidelines (see below). Admission is required for patients with malignant hypertension, ie if the patient is showing signs of encephalopathy (headache, focal central nervous system (CNS) signs, papilloedema, drowsiness, blurred vision).

INITIAL MANAGEMENT

When a diagnosis has been established, all hypertensive patients should have the following investigations:

- Urea and electrolytes (U&Es)

- Fasting lipid profile

- Fasting glucose

- Urine dipstick analysis for protein and blood (to exclude renal disease)

- ECG (echo is indicated if there are ECG signs of left ventricular hypertrophy).

Stop any medication that might make the BP worse, eg anti-inflammatories, steroids and the oral contraceptive pill. Lifestyle interventions are vital for everybody: exercise, smoking cessation, weight loss and a low-salt diet.

TREATMENT TARGETS

For most patients over the age of 50, systolic BP is more important than diastolic BP in terms of risk of CVD.

- **In non-diabetic patients, the aim is to reduce the BP to below 140/85 mmHg.** The maximum acceptable level (audit standard) is **150/90 mmHg.**

- **In diabetic patients, patients with established CVD and patients with renal impairment, BP should be reduced to below 130/80 mmHg.** The maximum acceptable level is **140/80 mmHg.**

NOTE: These values are based on clinic readings. Targets for ambulatory BP readings and home readings should be adjusted downwards by 10/5 mmHg. Therefore, compared to the clinic target of 140/85 mmHg, average home readings and ambulatory BP readings should be <130/80 mmHg (with average night-time BP <120/70 mmHg and average daytime BP <135/85 mmHg for ambulatory readings).

WHAT MEDICATION TO USE?

This is where it gets confusing! The National Institute for Clinical Excellence (NICE) and the BHS offer different guidance on initial treatment. NICE suggests the initial use of a thiazide diuretic for all patients over the age of 55 (except those with gout, unless covered with allopurinol); this is based mainly on the large ALLHAT study, which was carried out in the USA (*Journal of the American Medical Association* 2002; **288**: 2981–2997). However, critics of the ALLHAT study claim that it cannot be applied to the UK population, because a large percentage of trial patients (35%) were Afro-Caribbean, and this group responds particularly well to diuretics.

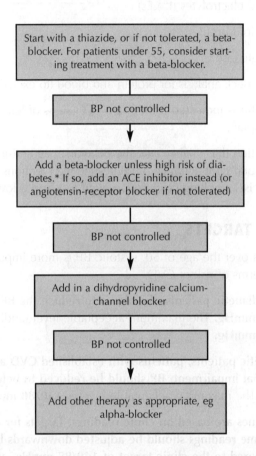

*Patients at high risk of diabetes:

- Strong family history of diabetes
- Impaired glucose tolerance
- Fasting glucose >6.5 mmol/l
- Clinically obese with body mass index (BMI) >30 kg/m^2
- South Asians and Afro-Caribbeans.

Figure 1.1 NICE guidance (recommended by most Primary Care Organisations). ACE, angiotensin-converting enzyme.

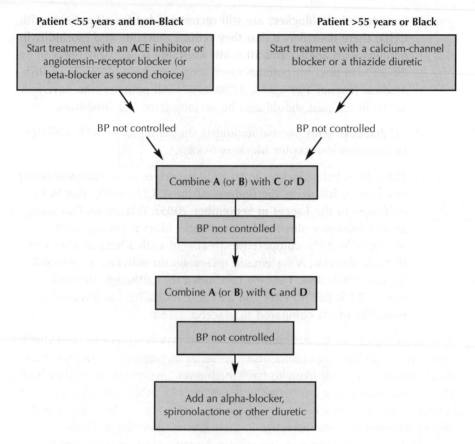

Figure 1.2 BHS guidance: 'ABCD' (with copyright permission from the British Hypertension Society, 'Recommendations for combining blood pressure lowering drugs/ABCD rule', *Journal of Human Hypertension*, 2004, 18, p.150, figure 3)

NOTE:

1 There is strong evidence to support the BHS guidelines when treating Black patients; in most studies, beta-blockers and angiotensin-converting enzyme (ACE) inhibitors have been shown to be of no benefit in treating this group (*Annals of Internal Medicine* 2004; 141: 614–627; *Effective Health Care* 2004; 8(4)).

2 The full benefit to be gained from any BP-lowering medication will take about 4 weeks to achieve. If after 4 weeks BP control is still suboptimal, the dose of the medication should be titrated up (except for thiazides, which are not more effective at higher doses, but may cause more side-effects). After this, it is reasonable either to change to an alternative treatment (if the hypertension is mild), or to add in a new drug.

3 Long-term beta-blockers are still recommended for all patients with CHD; there is evidence that they reduce mortality and morbidity in patients with angina and after MI. Mortality is probably reduced by 20–25% in post-MI patients given long-term beta-blockade (*British Medical Journal* 1999; 318: 1730–1737). All patients who have had an MI in the past should also be on long-term ACE inhibitors.

4 All diabetics with microalbuminuria should be on an ACE inhibitor or angiotensin-receptor blockers (ARBs).

5 The role of beta-blockers in treating hypertension is currently being questioned, following the findings of the ASCOT study (due to be published in the *Lancet* in September 2005). This shows that using an ACE inhibitor plus a calcium channel blocker cuts all cause mortality by 15% compared to treatment with a beta-blocker and thiazide diuretic. A systematic review on the efficiacy of atenolol (*Lancet* 2004; 364: 1684–9) concluded that although atenolol lowers BP, it has no effect on all cause mortality, cardiovascular mortality or MI compared to placebo.

The rationale behind the BHS guidelines is that hypertension can be divided into two categories: 'high renin' and 'low renin' hypertension. Younger, non-Black patients are more likely to have 'high renin' hypertension; studies have shown that renin levels are higher in young people and in white people. ACE inhibitors and beta-blockers both inhibit the renin–angiotensin system, and should therefore be more effective in these patient groups. NICE does not support the BHS because there have been no large randomised controlled trials yet to validate this approach, and thiazide diuretics are much cheaper than other antihypertensive drug groups. The cost issue is a debatable one however, in that it is likely that a higher percentage of patients will achieve optimal BP control with only one agent if the BHS advice is followed, compared with NICE guidance.

CAUTIONS

- Don't use a thiazide diuretic in patients who suffer from gout, as it may precipitate an attack.

- ACE inhibitors and ARBs should not usually be used in patients with moderate to severe aortic stenosis (if the gradient is >64 mmHg). These drugs can exacerbate symptoms, but usually do so quickly if they are going to have an adverse effect at all; cardiologists will sometimes introduce them cautiously if there is concomitant left ventricular dysfunction.

- ACE inhibitors can worsen renal function in patients with renal artery stenosis.

- Don't use beta-blockers in asthmatics, and use them with caution in patients with peripheral artery disease and chronic obstructive pulmonary disease (COPD). Patients whose COPD shows little or no reversibility with beta-agonists (eg those with emphysema) will probably be able to tolerate beta-blockers; in this case, a very low dose of a cardioselective drug should be used.

- Cardioselective beta-blockers (eg carvedilol and bisoprolol) are preferable for patients with heart failure, but should be introduced very gradually, probably under specialist supervision.

- Adding a thiazide to a beta-blocker in patients at high risk of developing diabetes is not recommended by the BHS or by NICE; the LIFE trial (*Lancet* 2002; **359**: 995) demonstrated a 15% excess risk of new-onset type 2 diabetes over 5 years with this combination compared with an ARB used with a thiazide diuretic. Indapamide has a more favourable effect on glucose than bendroflumethiazide, but is several times more expensive. Patients receiving beta-blockers, even when used alone, are more likely to develop diabetes than patients on ACE inhibitors or ARBs.

- Extreme caution should be used if combining verapamil or diltiazem with a beta-blocker, because the patient might be tipped into heart failure. Long-acting dihydropyridine calcium-channel blockers (eg amlodipine and felodipine) should be safe in combination with a beta-blocker, but are more likely to cause ankle swelling than diltiazem or verapamil. Short-acting calcium-channel blockers should also be used with caution when combined with a beta-blocker.

MEASURING U&ES IN PATIENTS ON ACE INHIBITORS

Patients who have a normal baseline creatinine and who do not have significant co-morbidities are at low risk of suffering from renal impairment while on an ACE inhibitor. In these patients, the following measurements should be made:

- Baseline U&Es

- A single U&E check while the dose is being titrated up

- An annual U&E check.

This only applies to patients with normal renal function, which does not deteriorate after the initial introduction of an ACE inhibitor; others will need to be monitored more closely. ACE inhibitors should be withdrawn if the creatinine rises by >50% of its baseline value, or exceeds 200 µmol/l; whichever is less.

HYPERTENSION IN THE ELDERLY

About 70% of people over the age of 60 in the UK have a BP of >140/90 mmHg. Elderly people are likely to benefit from blood pressure lowering as much as, if not more than, younger patients in terms of lowering their cerebrovascular accident (CVA) risk. Treatment can certainly be continued beyond the age of 80 for anyone at significant risk of CVD, particularly if they are otherwise well and do not suffer from adverse effects because of the medication. However, it should be remembered that there is little trial evidence supporting the use of antihypertensive treatment in the over-85 age group, and the risk of falls from postural hypotension should not be underestimated; mortality after a fractured neck of femur is very high. Thiazide diuretics and calcium-channel blockers are likely to be most effective in the elderly.

GENERAL MEDICAL SERVICES (GMS) CONTRACT AND HYPERTENSION

In order to be awarded the maximum number of quality points, practices must achieve the following standards:

- There must be a record of the BP of at least 55% of over-45-year-old patients within the past 5 years (the under-45s are not mentioned); this is in order for the practice to be awarded extra organisational indicator points.

- There should be a register in place for patients with established hypertension.

- 90% of hypertensive patients should have had their smoking status recorded at least once and 90% of smokers should have been given smoking cessation advice.

- 90% of hypertensive patients should have had a BP recorded within the past 9 months.

- 70% of hypertensive patients should have a BP of ≤150/90 mmHg (this must be the last recorded reading, which must have been done within the past 9 months).

- At least 55% of diabetic patients should have a BP of ≤145/85 mmHg (using the last recorded reading).

ANTIPLATELET THERAPY

ASPIRIN

This should be prescribed at a dose of 75 mg/day for:

- Anyone with hypertension over the age of 50 with a CVD risk of >20% over 10 years

- Anyone over 50 with diabetes

- Anyone over 50 with target organ damage (eg LVH or renal impairment)

- Anyone with established CVD

DIPYRIDAMOLE

The combination of modified-release dipyridamole and aspirin is recommended by NICE for 2 years after an ischaemic CVA or transient ischaemic attack (TIA). After this, the patient can revert back to using aspirin alone. The dose of dipyridamole should usually be titrated up to 200 mg bd over the course of 2 weeks. Headache is a common side-effect.

Dipyridamole can be used as an alternative to aspirin for patients who are intolerant of the latter; it should usually be prescribed before clopidogrel in this case.

CLOPIDOGREL

Clopidogrel should be prescribed in the following circumstances:

- For patients requiring anti-platelet treatment who are intolerant of aspirin and dipyridamole.

- In combination with aspirin for up to 12 months following non-ST segment elevation acute coronary syndrome or unstable angina.

- For the first 2 years following an MI of a diagnosis of peripheral arterial disease in patients who are aspirin intolerant (ie in preference to dipyridamole.

CHOLESTEROL-LOWERING

Risk charts are designed to allow a CVD risk to be calculated for each individual patient; this is useful when considering whether to start someone on BP- or cholesterol-lowering treatment.

The Joint British Society charts are the ones recommended by BHS and they have been updated recently to reflect CVD risk rather than CHD risk (see below), on the basis of evidence from several new trials. They are, however, still derived from the Framingham data, collected from a cohort of 5000 people from North America who were followed up for 10 years. Diabetes has now been removed as an extra risk factor, because most diabetics automatically qualify for treatment with statins. The charts are only intended to be used for primary prevention. There are just three age bands (<50, 50–60 and >60) in the new charts, which means that anyone under 50 will be considered to be the same age (ie 49) for the purposes of assessing cardiovascular risk.

Figure 1.3 New Joint British Society CVD risk charts (with copyright permission from the British Hypertension Society, 'Joint British Societies CVD Risk Prediction Chart,' *Journal of Human Hypertension*, 2004, 18, 149–150, figure 2)

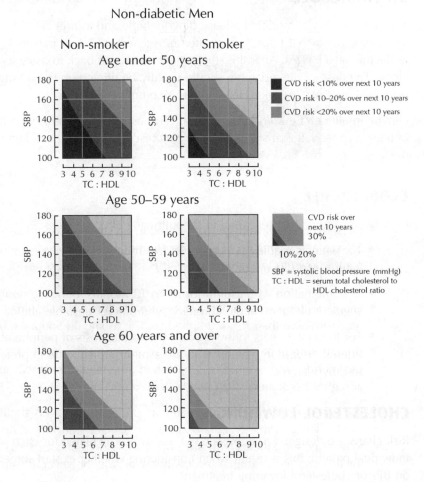

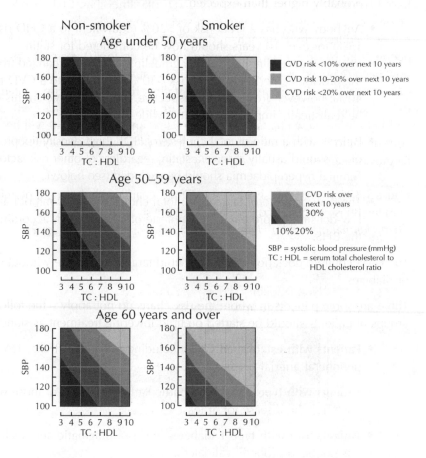

- Ex-smokers should still be considered to be smokers for at least 5 years after giving up (it is a minimum of 10 years before the risk comes down to the same level as it is for someone who has never smoked).

- People with a strong family history of premature CVD should probably have their risk multiplied by 1.5, as should South Asians.

- Patients with impaired glucose tolerance, patients with raised triglycerides and women who have had a premature menopause are at higher risk than is suggested by the charts.

- For hypertensive patients on treatment, pretreatment levels should be used where possible when assessing risk. Clinical judgement needs to be used for patients who have been well controlled for years and for whom a pre-treatment level is not available; however, if using treatment BP levels, bear in mind that the patient's CVD risk is probably higher than expected.

- Anybody who has a CVD risk of >20% (equivalent to a CHD risk of 15%) for over 10 years should now be considered for statin treatment according to the BHS guidelines. This has changed from the previous criterion of CHD risk >30% (equivalent to a CVD risk of 40%); however, from a cost perspective, it is unclear when this could be realistically implemented nationwide.

- Patients with a ratio of total cholesterol:HDL (high-density lipoprotein) of >7 should usually receive a statin, regardless of other risk factors. Familial hyperlipidaemia should be excluded (see below).

- The new cholesterol targets are: total cholesterol <4.0 mmol/l and low-density lipoprotein (LDL) cholesterol <2.0 mmol/l, according to the BHS.

The GMS contract does not specify any lipid targets for people without CVD or diabetes.

There are some patients in whom the risk charts do not apply – the following groups of patients should be started on lipid-lowering treatment as standard:

- **Patients with established CVD** (including ischaemic stroke, TIA and peripheral arterial disease).

- **Patients with type 2 diabetes** (particularly if >50 and/or those who have had the disease for at least 10 years).

- **Patients >40 with type 1 diabetes** (this is a pragmatic approach that has not been properly validated).

HDL

HDL is cardioprotective, and having a low level (of <1 mmol/l in men and <1.2 mmol/l in women) is a strong, independent risk factor for CHD. To boost HDL levels, patients should be encouraged to exercise and to stop smoking. Drinking moderate amounts of alcohol and eating oily fish at least twice a week (in particular mackerel, sardines and herring) can also increase HDL.

FAMILIAL HYPERLIPIDAEMIA

The charts do not apply in patients with familial hyperlipidaemia. Familial hyperlipidaemia should be suspected in patients with a total cholesterol of >7.5 mmol/l who have a strong family history of CHD. They may or may not have physical signs such as corneal arcus or tendon xanthomata (found commonly on the extensor tendons of the hands, the patellar tendon and the Achilles tendon). There are many different types of familial hyperlipidaemia, and often environmental factors such as obesity play as large a part in subsequent morbidity as do genetic factors. The most common types encountered in general practice are:

- **Familial combined hyperlipidaemia (incidence 1:200).** The patient will have raised total cholesterol, LDL and/or triglycerides. HDL is often low and apoprotein B is elevated. Physical signs are quite rare. There is a big overlap between this condition and the metabolic syndrome, with insulin resistance occurring in both. The cause is poorly understood and diagnosis is difficult. Complicated genetic factors seem to interact with environmental factors to produce morbidity. Often, CHD does not occur until a patient is in their 50s or 60s. Statin treatment is not initially mandatory; see below.

- **Polygenic hypercholesterolaemia (incidence 1:250).** The patient usually has a cholesterol of >7.5 mmol/l, with raised LDL. They will probably not have physical signs. Again, environmental factors are important and statin treatment may not always be necessary.

- **Familial hypercholesterolaemia (incidence of heterozygotes 1:500, homozygotes 1:1 000 000).** The genetics of this condition are more straightforward; it is an autosomal dominant condition. Physical signs are common. Cholesterol is raised from birth and a fatal MI can occur in the patient's 20s or 30s. Statin treatment is essential.

Patients with polygenic hyperlipidaemias may not always need statin treatment, and can sometimes respond to lifestyle modifications. However, if they do not, treatment for CVD risk factors should be initiated sooner rather than later, in order to prevent premature cardiovascular morbidity and mortality. Diagnosis usually relies on screening the patient's family and genetic testing is rarely helpful.

MONITORING STATINS

- There is no need to monitor patients on 10 mg simvastatin.

- All other patients should have baseline liver function tests (LFTs), which should be repeated 1–3 months after treatment is initiated.

- Thereafter, LFTs should be checked at intervals of 6 months for the first year of treatment, and then annually.

ANGINA MANAGEMENT

GENERAL MANAGEMENT

All risk factors should be targeted, including lipid levels, smoking, obesity, inactivity and raised blood pressure. Patients should be screened for diabetes, and a statin initiated if cholesterol is greater than 3.5 mmol/l and BP reduced to ≤130/80 mmHg. Aspirin should be given prophylactically to all angina sufferers, or dipyridamole if aspirin is not tolerated. Patients should be investigated for anaemia and thyroid disfunction.

SPECIFIC DRUG TREATMENT OF ANGINA

- Sublingual glyceryl trinitrate (GTN) is the best first-line treatment for an acute angina attack. Patients with normal or low blood pressure should be warned to sit down before taking it, in case they feel dizzy.

- Beta-blockers are the cornerstone of therapy and should always be prescribed for angina sufferers unless there is a contraindication; the dose should be increased to the maximum tolerated. There is definite evidence of the benefit of long-term beta-blockade post-MI in terms of morbidity and mortality and, logically, this benefit should also extend to angina patients. Beta-blockers are also effective in reducing angina symptoms. (IMAGE study. *J Am Coll Cardiol* 1996, 27: 311–6.) Beta-blockers should not be stopped suddenly, they should be tailed off over a period of 4 weeks.

- Rate-limiting calcium-channel blockers such as diltiazem and verapamil are alternative choices for patients intolerant of beta-blockers. Dihydropyridine calcium-channel blockers (eg amlodipine, nifedipine and felodipine) are useful when given in combination with beta-blockers if extra medication is needed to achieve symptom control. Calcium-channel blockers have not been proved to have a beneficial effect on mortality, but are useful for preventing angina.

- Oral nitrates are effective in preventing symptoms, but the patient should have at least 12 nitrate-free hours each day to prevent tolerance. Isosorbide mononitrate (ISMN) can be given in conjunction with beta-blockers or calcium-channel blockers to achieve better symptom control.

- Nicorandil is a potassium-channel activator, and is increasingly being used as the next step after beta-blockers, usually at a dose of 20 mg bd.

The precise role of ACE inhibitors in treating patients with angina is yet to be clarified. Data from the HOPE study (NEJM 2000; 342: 145–53) and EUROPA study (Lancet 2003; 362: 782) suggest a small additional benefit of ACE inhibition in treating patients with stable coronary artery disease.

GMS CONTRACT AND CHD

In order to be awarded maximum quality points, practices must achieve the following standards:

- There must be a register of patients with CHD.

- 90% of patients with angina diagnosed after April 2003 should have had an exercise test or specialist assessment.

- 90% of CHD patients should have had their smoking status recorded within the past 15 months (except those who have never smoked, in which case a single recording is sufficient); 70% of smokers with CHD should have had smoking cessation advice within the past 15 months.

- 90% of patients with CHD should have had a BP recording done within the past 15 months.

- At least 70% of CHD patients should have their BP controlled to ≤150/90 mmHg.

- 90% of CHD patients should have had their cholesterol checked in the past 15 months and this should be ≤5 mmol/l in 60% of people.

- 90% of CHD patients should be on aspirin or equivalent.

- 50% of CHD patients should be on a beta-blocker (unless there is a specific contraindication).

- 70% of post-MI patients (diagnosed after April 2003) should be on an ACE inhibitor.

- 85% of CHD patients should have a record of influenza immunisation in the preceding year.

PERIPHERAL ARTERY DISEASE (PAD)

Again, all risk factors should be targeted, with similar reductions in cholesterol and BP being aimed for. ACE inhibitors may be beneficial, even apart from their antihypertensive effect and should be used as first-line agents in all patients with PAD, regardless of their BP. All patients with PAD should also be offered a statin.

Diabetes should be excluded; 20% of patients with vascular claudication are diabetic. Smoking cessation is vital. Aspirin should be prescribed prophylactically.

The drug **cilostazol** has been found to increase walking distance in patients with claudication.

CVA MANAGEMENT: NATIONAL CLINICAL GUIDELINES FOR STROKE (JUNE 2004)

Patients who have had a CVA have a 30–43% risk of having another stroke within 5 years. TIA patients have a 20% risk of having a full CVA within the first month. Aggressive control of risk factors is therefore very important, BP being the most important one.

- All patients with acute CVA should be referred to hospital (patients treated on a stroke unit have an improved prognosis). In the case of a TIA, outpatient review should take place within 7 days. However, if the patient has more than one TIA in the same week, they should be admitted to hospital. Current stroke guidelines state that CVA patients should have a brain scan within 24 hours, although this does not apply to TIA patients.

- CVA (with ischaemic aetiology) and TIA patients should receive 300 mg aspirin as soon as possible after their symptoms have stabilised, and certainly within 48 hours. This is often prescribed in hospital if the patient is going to be admitted. If not – for example in the case of a TIA – it should be prescribed in the community. A haemorrhagic stroke should be suspected in the following cases:

    1   If the patient is on anticoagulants.

    2   There is a known bleeding tendency.

    3   The patient has a depressed level of consciousness.

    4   The patient has unexplained progressive or fluctuating symptoms.

    5   The patient has papilloedema, neck stiffness or fever.

    6   The patient describes a severe headache before the onset of symptoms.

- A few centres offer thrombolysis for ischaemic CVA; this must be given within 6 hours of the onset of symptoms, and only after the patient has had a CT scan of the brain.

- After the initial dose of 300 mg, aspirin should be continued at a dose of 75 mg per day, sometimes in combination with modified-release dipyridamole 200 mg bd for the first 2 years (as per NICE guidance). Dipyridamole should be started at a low dose and then increased over 2 weeks, in order to reduce side-effects.

- Dipyridamole alone or clopidogrel alone can be used in aspirin-intolerant patients (according to NICE, dipyridamole should be tried first).

- Lower BP to ≤140/85 mmHg (or to 130/80 mmHg in diabetic patients). This should only be done in the acute phase if there are likely to be complications from hypertension, eg hypertensive encephalopathy. If not, patients should have their BP monitored, and hypertension persisting for more than 2 weeks should be treated. Some centres have stricter BP criteria of 130/80 mmHg for all patients: in a sense, the lower the BP, the less likely the patient is to have a recurrence and there is no evidence of a 'J-shaped curve'. Thiazides and/or ACE inhibitors are usually recommended, even if the patient is normotensive and, in this case, BP should be reduced to the lowest level that the patient can tolerate.

- All CVA and TIA patients with a cholesterol of >3.5 mmol/l should be offered a statin unless contraindicated. This is in order to reduce the risk of a further CVA, but also to reduce the risk of MI; most patients who have had a CVA have a ≥30% 10-year risk of CHD.

- Check for atrial fibrillation and, if present, consider warfarinisation.

- Arrange a carotid ultrasound; endarterectomy is more beneficial if done within 12 weeks of a TIA. The number of patients you need to treat in order to save one life is approximately 26. (Cochrane Library Issue 1, 2004).

- Other lifestyle factors are, as usual, very important: smoking (quality points are given for recording this information and giving smoking cessation advice), obesity, lack of exercise, salt in the diet (limit to <6 g/day), etc.

- Depression is common in CVA patients; it is always a good idea to screen for this.

GMS CONTRACT AND CEREBROVASCULAR DISEASE

In order to be awarded maximum quality points, practices must achieve the following standards:

- There must be a register of all patients with stroke or TIA.

- At least 80% of patients who have had a CVA after April 2003 should have been referred for a CT brain scan to confirm the diagnosis.

- 90% of patients should have had their smoking status recorded within the past 15 months (except for people who have never smoked, when a single recording will suffice) and 70% of smokers should have been offered smoking cessation advice.

- The BP should have been recorded at least once in the past 15 months in 90% of patients.

- 70% of patients should have a BP of <150/90 mmHg.

- 90% of patients should have had their cholesterol checked in the past 15 months and this should be ≤5 mmol/l in 60% of people.

- 90% of patients with non-haemorrhagic CVA should be on aspirin or an equivalent.

- 85% of patients should have a record of influenza immunisation in the preceding year.

HEART FAILURE

The median age at diagnosis is 76. The incidence overall is approximately 0.9/1000 per year, but is much higher in the over-85 age group (approaching 1% per annum). NICE updated their guidance in 2003 and the following section is based on these guidelines.

DIAGNOSIS

A diagnosis can be made on the basis of ECG and B-type natriuretic peptide (BNP) tests. BNP is a highly sensitive test, and if it is negative the patient can be reassured that they do not have heart failure (Table 1.2). It is not particularly specific however, so people who test positive do not necessarily have left ventricular dysfunction (LVD), but should be referred for echocardiography to confirm the diagnosis.

BNP measurement is not available to all GPs; in this case, referral for echo should be based on ECG findings. Patients with LVD will usually have ECG abnormalities, eg left ventricular hypertrophy. Patients who have a normal echo, but clinically still have symptoms of heart failure, may have diastolic dysfunction. They should be referred to a specialist for diagnosis.

Other recommended investigations are: chest X-ray (CXR), spirometry (to exclude a respiratory problem) and baseline blood tests (full blood count (FBC), U&Es, lipids, glucose, thyroid function tests (TFTs)).

BNP value (ng/l)	Interpretation
<50 in young people or <100 in the elderly	Heart failure excluded
100–600	Borderline
>600	Heart failure very likely

Table 1.2: Interpretation of the BNP test

TREATMENT

Lifestyle measures are vital: smoking cessation, a low-salt and low-fat diet, alcohol reduction and exercise training. Alcohol-induced cardiac failure is more common than most people realise, and patients should always be asked about their intake. Medication should be reviewed and stopped if it is likely to be making the LVD worse (eg non-steroidal anti-inflammatory drugs (NSAIDs), lithium, steroids). If the patient cannot do without an NSAID, it is better that they are on a low dose of ibuprofen than other, more cardiotoxic, drugs such as diclofenac or indometacin. Valvular heart disease (eg aortic stenosis) can result in cardiac failure and is potentially reversible. Drug treatment improves morbidity and mortality in LVD and should be initiated as follows:

- **Aspirin** (75 mg/day).

- **ACE inhibitors and ARBs**: these should be started off at a low dose and titrated upwards. U&Es need to be checked about 1 week after treatment is started. ACE inhibitors are usually used as first-line treatment, and an ARB is substituted if the patient is intolerant; the CHARM alternative (*Lancet* 2003; **362**: 759–781) and VALIANT (*New England Journal of Medicine* 2003; **349**: 20) trials have shown that ARBs are also effective in heart failure. The ACE inhibitor dose should be doubled at intervals of at least 2 weeks, aiming for the target dose for LVD (eg lisinopril 30 mg od, ramipril 10 mg od or enalapril 20 mg bd). Rises in creatinine of 50% from the baseline value or up to 200 mmol/l (whichever is smaller) are acceptable. There is a huge amount of trial data supporting the use of ACE inhibitors in heart failure (eg 'Consensus', *NEJM* 1987; 316: 1429–35 and 'Solv'd' *NEJM* 1991; 325: 293–302)

- **Beta-blockers**: only the selective beta-blockers, bisoprolol, metoprolol and carvedilol have been used in the big heart failure trials ('CIBIS II', *Lancet*, 1999; 353: 9–13 and 'MERIT-HF', Lancet 1999; 353: 2001–7, and 'Copernicus', *NEJM* 2001; 344: 1651–8 and 'BEST', *NEJM* 2001; 344: 1659–67) and it is one of these three which will normally be initiated for heart failure. However, if a patient is already on a non-selective beta-blocker prior to their diagnosis, they can continue on it. Beta-blockers should be introduced very cautiously, starting off with a low dose (1.25 mg od for bisoprolol and 3.125 mg bd for carvedilol) and titrating upwards over several weeks; the dose should be doubled at intervals of no less than 2 weeks, until target therapeutic doses are reached, and the patient should be warned that they might initially feel worse. Beta-blockers should only be introduced once the patient is stabilised on their final dosage of ACE inhibitor. Only patients with stable heart failure should be tried on beta-blockers; these drugs should never be introduced in patients with worsening symptoms.

- **Diuretics** produce significant functional improvement. Impact on mortality and general prognosis is not known. They should be used as a matter of course, to help with symptoms of breathlessness. Diuretics are less helpful in patients with diastolic dysfunction.

- **Spironolactone** may decrease mortality if used in addition to the above treatments, at a dose of 25 mg od ('RALES trial', *Lancet,* 1999; 341: 709–17). Hyperkalaemia and renal impairment are possible, and potassium levels should be carefully monitored.

- **Digoxin** can be started in any patients with LVD and concomitant atrial fibrillation. It can also be used in patients in sinus rhythm as an adjunct to ACE inhibitors, diuretics and beta-blockers if necessary.

DIASTOLIC DYSFUNCTION

Patients with a normal ejection fraction on echo may still have diastolic dysfunction; this should be suspected if the history is suggestive of heart failure and other diagnoses such as COPD and dyspnoea due to obesity have been excluded. These patients are often hypertensive, but may not complain of very much peripheral oedema. In general, diastolic dysfunction is a less serious disease than LVD and is less likely to result in admission. Patients should be treated in a similar way, but rarely benefit much from diuretics because they are not usually oedematous.

GMS CONTRACT AND LVD

Maximum quality points are awarded to practices who achieve the following standards:

- A register of patients with CHD and LVD.

- Echocardiographical confirmation in 90% of their LVD cases diagnosed after April 2003 (in patients with concomitant CHD only).

- At least 70% of patients with LVD and CHD should be prescribed ACE inhibitors or ARBs.

ATRIAL FIBRILLATION

Rate control is at least as important as rhythm control in atrial fibrillation ('Affirm' study. *New England Journal of Medicine* 2002; **347**: 1825), so a medication such as a beta-blocker, a rate-limiting calcium-channel blocker or digoxin that slows the pulse rate should be considered. Untreated atrial fibrillation is a strong risk factor for CVA, with an incidence of approximately 5% per year overall.

Patients with the following risk factors are at moderate or high risk of having an adverse outcome from untreated atrial fibrillation and should be considered for anticoagulation with warfarin:

- Previous history of CVA or TIA (very high risk – should definitely receive warfarin).

- Hypertension, LVF or diabetes (high risk if >65 – should definitely receive warfarin; moderate risk if <65 – consider warfarin).

- >65 years of age with no other risk factor (moderate risk – consider warfarin).

If high-risk patients are deemed unsuitable for warfarinisation, they should receive high-dose aspirin 300 mg od(/).

Patients who are over 65 without additional risk factors and those under 65 with co-existent diabetes, CHD or hypertension should be offered a choice between warfarin and aspirin. Patients under 65 with no additional risk factors should be given aspirin at a dose of 75–150 mg per day.

CHAPTER 2
DEMENTIA

CHAPTER 2
DEMENTIA

DEMENTIA

The three most common causes of dementia in the UK are Alzheimer's disease (AD; accounts for 55% of cases), vascular dementia (25%) and Lewy body dementia (10–15%). Alzheimer's disease is characterised by a long preclinical period during which subtle cognitive deficits are often detectable, although the patient may not always report subjective memory loss. Preclinical deficits have been shown in global indicators of cognition, such as the mini mental state examination and in specific tests that assess psychomotor speed, attention, verbal ability and visuospatial skill. However, these tests are often not very specific and may also be positive in patients with mild age-related memory loss.

Vascular dementia commonly shows a more 'step-wise' progression than AD, with sudden, acute deteriorations resulting from ischaemic events. Risk factors for CVD should be addressed in these patients.

It can be difficult to distinguish between age-associated cognitive changes and early dementia. Patients with memory loss are at greater risk of developing dementia. If the family report subtle personality changes or language difficulties (a classic example being the inability to interpret proverbs), dementia is more likely. Various different terms have been used to describe memory problems in the elderly. Examples are:

- **Age-associated memory impairment**. This is very common in the over-65 age group, affecting up to 40% of people; the patients themselves complain of subjective memory impairment and they perform less well on standardised objective memory tests than younger adults. Age-associated memory impairment can almost be considered to be a variant of normal and only 1% of these people go on to develop AD per year. There is some evidence that ginkgo biloba (at doses of 120–240 mg tds of standardised extract) protects against memory loss (Cochrane Library, Issue 2, Oxford 2003).

- **Mild cognitive impairment (MCI)**. This affects 10% of the over-65 age group. Memory loss is more marked, and is similar to that found in early AD; indeed, distinguishing between these two conditions can be difficult. Approximately 12% of patients with MCI develop AD per year and ideally the patient should be followed up twice a year to check for this.

DIAGNOSIS

AD cannot be accurately diagnosed on the basis of cognitive function tests alone; these tests must be used in conjunction with a full history from the patient and their carers. Screening blood tests are important, to exclude any reversible causes of dementia and should include FBC, U&Es, LFTs, TFTs, vitamin B12, folate, syphilis serology and glucose. Brain imaging is usually performed as well, although this may lead to over-diagnosis of vascular dementia as a result of discovering incidental evidence of mild age-related ischaemic events.

The 30-point mini mental state examination (MMSE) is the most frequently used test to detect cognitive impairment (see page 33). However, there are problems with sensitivity and specificity; for example, many highly educated patients score better than expected. As an approximate guide, scores on the MMSE of between 21 and 26 may indicate mild AD; scores between 10 and 20, moderate AD; and a score of <10 is usually indicative of severe AD.

There are several newer alternatives to the MMSE. An example is the DemTect®, which is a new, highly sensitive psychometric screening test used to identify patients with MCI and early dementia. It comprises of five tasks: a word list, a number transcoding task, a word fluency task, digit span reverse, and delayed recall of the word list. The DemTect® appears to be superior to the MMSE in detecting MCI and AD patients, with sensitivities of 80% and 100%, respectively (*International Journal of Geriatric Psychiatry* 2004; 19 (2): 136). It is short (8–10 minutes), easy to administer, and scoring (out of a maximum of 18) is independent of age and education. It helps to determine whether cognitive performance is adequate for age (13–18 points), or whether MCI (9–12 points) or dementia (8 points or below) should be suspected.

WHEN TO REFER?

Because of the difficulties in coming to a definite diagnosis, the question of when to refer is often problematic for the GP. Early diagnosis is important, as the patient will then have the opportunity to make plans for their future, and to consider whether they wish to prepare an advance directive. Also, if treatment with cholinesterase inhibitors is to be considered, this is better done early on in the course of the illness. In general, patients who score less than 24 on the MMSE should probably be referred. Screening blood tests as detailed above should usually be carried out in primary care.

DRUG TREATMENT FOR ALZHEIMER'S DISEASE

The future of the cholinesterase inhibitors and memantine is looking uncertain at present. The government has opposed recent NICE draft guidance in which these drugs are no longer recommended for newly diagnosed patients with AD. NICE 2001 guidance states that the cholinesterase inhibitors can be used in the treatment of AD, as long as initiation takes place in a specialist clinic and is discontinued if the MMSE deteriorates or drops to <12.

The latest NICE draft guidance was informed by several studies, including the AD 2000 trial (Lancet 2004; 363: 2105-15) which showed that donepezil does not delay entry into institutional care, progression of disability or improve behavioural or psychological symptoms. However, political pressures may mean that this new guidance is not implemented.

HELPING PATIENTS TO REMAIN AT HOME

There are many different devices available to help patients with mild dementia to continue living in their own homes safely. Examples include plugs to prevent the bath from overflowing, passive infrared lights and switches, automatic shut-off devices for ovens, pill boxes fitted with alarms, passive personal alarm devices (activated as a result of inactivity) and electronic calendars that indicate what day and date it is. The Disabled Living Foundation can demonstrate available equipment and discuss options with the patient or their carers (see Useful Contact Information for further details). The Enable Project website (www.enableproject.org) explains how to purchase this equipment.

DRUG TREATMENT FOR DISRUPTIVE FEATURES IN DEMENTIA

Patients with advanced dementia may become increasingly aggressive or agitated. Symptoms that are present for more than 3 months are likely persist long term. Sometimes simple measures can help, such as, avoiding unfamiliar surroundings and people. Some patients respond well to soothing music or to aromatherapy. Unaddressed pain or physical discomfort may result in deterioration; easily reversible causes such as chronic constipation should not be overlooked. Hearing and visual loss should also be corrected as far as possible.

Sedative medication is often prescribed because it makes life easier for the patient's carers; unfortunately, it is rarely in the best interests of the patient to be sedated and most of the available drugs have significant side-effects. In March 2004, the Committee on Safety of Medicines (CSM) issued a warning about using atypical antipsychotics such as risperidone and olanzapine in patients with dementia; their use appears to be associated with a threefold increase in the risk of CVA. Although this risk has only been demonstrated with risperidone and olanzapine, it may also apply to other atypical antipsychotics. The CSM recommendations are listed below:

- Risperidone or olanzapine should not be used for the treatment of behavioural symptoms of dementia.

- Use of risperidone for the management of acute psychotic conditions in elderly patients who also have dementia should be limited to the short term and should be guided by specialist advice (olanzapine is not licensed for management of acute psychoses).

- Prescribers should consider carefully the risk of cerebrovascular events before treating any patient with a previous history of stroke or transient ischaemic attack with atypical antipsychotics. Consideration should also be given to other risk factors for cerebrovascular disease, including hypertension, diabetes, current smoking and atrial fibrillation.

Other potential treatment options include the conventional antipsychotics, such as chlorpromazine (at doses of about 75 mg daily), benzodiazepines (not recommended for long-term use), antidepressants and carbamazepine (at doses of 300 mg daily). There is only limited evidence supporting the use of carbamazepine, and treatment benefits will probably take at least 3 weeks to become apparent. There is some evidence that conventional antipsychotics are no safer than atypical antipsychotics in terms of CVA risk (BMJ 2005; 330: 445-8), and guidance may change in the future.

MINI MENTAL STATE EXAMINATION

- What day of the week is it? (1 point)

- What is the date today? (3 points, 1 each for day, month and year)

- What is the season? (1 point)

- Can you tell me where we are now? (1 point)

- What are two main streets nearby? (1 point)

- What floor of the building are we on? (1 point)

- What is the address of the place where we are now? (1 point)

- Offer the patient a piece of paper on which is written the following, 'I am going to give you a piece of paper. When I do, take the paper in your right hand. Fold the paper in half with both hands and put the paper down in your lap.' (3 points, 1 for each action)

- Show the patient an everyday object, such as a pencil, and ask what it is called. (1 point)

- Show the patient another object, such as a wristwatch strap, and ask what it is called. (1 point)

- Say (once only), 'I am going to say something and I would like you to repeat it after me: "No ifs, ands or buts".' (1 point)

- Say, 'Please read what is written here and do what it says'. The card will say 'close your eyes.' (1 point if the action is carried out correctly)

- Say, 'Write a complete sentence on this sheet of paper'. The sentence must make sense and must contain a verb. (1 point)

- Say, 'Here is a drawing, please copy it.' The point is only given if the two shapes intersect to form a four-sided figure and all the angles are preserved. (1 point)

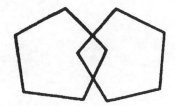

- Say, 'I am going to name three objects. After I have finished saying all three, I want you to repeat them. Try to remember what they are because I will ask you again in a few minutes.' Name three common objects, eg book, chair and pen. Score 1 point for each object if they are able to repeat it on the first attempt. (3 points)

- Say, 'Now I would like you to take 7 away from 100. Continue to take 7 away from your answer until I tell you to stop.' Carry on for five subtractions with one point scored each time a correct answer is given. (5 points)

- Say, 'What were the three objects I asked you to remember a few minutes ago?' Score 1 point for each correct answer. (3 points)

CHAPTER 3
DRIVER AND VEHICLE LICENSING AGENCY (DVLA) REGULATIONS

CHAPTER 3

DRIVER AND VEHICLE LICENSING AGENCY (DVLA) REGULATIONS

In general, the onus of responsibility lies with each individual to inform the DVLA if they are suffering from any clinical condition that might disqualify them from driving. It is the role of the GP to advise the patient that they may no longer be eligible to drive and to ask them to tell the DVLA. In rare circumstances, if the patient refuses to do this, the GP may be obliged to inform the DVLA on their behalf. The patient should be made aware that this might happen.

The DVLA will issue licences up to the age of 70. After this, they require confirmation from the patient that no medical disability is present. A 3-year licence will then be issued, which can be renewed.

COMMON MEDICAL CONDITIONS AFFECTING ELIGIBILITY TO DRIVE

(GROUP 1 REGULATIONS, IE TO DRIVE A PRIVATE VEHICLE)

- **Epilepsy.** The patient must have been seizure-free for 1 year from the date of the last attack, whether they were awake or asleep when it occurred. Exceptions are patients who have recently suffered a sleep attack but who have had no awake attacks for at least 3 years. This applies to partial and generalised seizures, as well as auras. Patients must attend for regular checks with their doctor and be compliant with treatment 'as far as practicable'. A licence is usually issued for 3 years. If the patient has only had one solitary fit (unprovoked by alcohol or drugs), they should have 1 year off driving, after which a full licence will be restored. Patients who have an isolated seizure after a head injury or CVA are not included in this category. In general, patients should be advised to refrain from driving for 6 months after anti-epileptic medication has been withdrawn, although this may not apply if they only suffer from sleep seizures.

- **Diabetes.** Insulin-treated diabetics must recognise warning symptoms of hypoglycaemia and meet the required visual standards. A 1-, 2- or 3-year licence will be issued. If the patient is only on temporary insulin treatment (up to 3 months), eg post-MI, then they may retain their licence, as long as they are not suffering from attacks of hypoglycaemia. Diabetics controlled on tablets should inform the DVLA, but may retain their licence until the age of 70 unless they develop specific complications such as retinopathy. Diet-controlled diabetics need not inform the DVLA.

- **CVA/TIA.** The patient should stop driving for at least 1 month, but may resume after this if clinical progress is satisfactory. The DVLA should only be informed if there is a residual neurological deficit after 1 month.

- **Serious head injury.** The patient will need 6–12 months off driving if there has been an acute intracerebral bleed requiring surgery, or a compound depressed skull fracture or dural tear with >24 hours post-traumatic amnesia. If there was loss of consciousness but no other complications, the patient need not inform the DVLA, providing recovery is complete.

- **CHD.** Patients who have uncontrolled angina must stop driving until their symptoms are adequately controlled. Driving must cease for at least 4 weeks following an acute MI or coronary artery bypass graft (CABG) and for 1 week after angioplasty. The DVLA need not be informed.

- **Deafness.** Patients need not notify the DVLA; their licence can be retained until the age of 70.

- **Alcohol misuse.** Persistent alcohol misuse, confirmed by medical enquiry and/or abnormal blood results (eg raised mean cell volume (MCV) or deranged LFTs), requires licence revocation until the patient has demonstrated that their drinking has been under control for at least 6 months, with normalisation of the blood tests. Alcoholic patients are required to be free from alcohol-related problems for at least 1 year, usually with complete abstinence and normalisation of blood results. In practice, it is difficult to determine whether a patient is merely misusing alcohol or is actually an alcoholic; the distinction between the two is often very blurred or non-existent. The license will be revoked for at least 1 year after an alcohol-related seizure.

- **Drug dependency.** Persistent use of cannabis leads to licence revocation until the patient has been free of use for at least 6 months. This period is extended to 1 year for other drugs, such as heroin, cocaine, morphine, benzodiazepines and methadone (unless the patient is on a consultant-supervised methadone maintenance programme and is fully compliant).

- **Visual disturbance.** The patient must be able to read a registration plate at a distance of 20 metres in good light, with the aid of glasses or contact lenses if necessary. Patients who lose vision in one eye must inform the DVLA. They can resume driving once they have adapted to their disability. Patients with visual field defects (eg homonymous hemianopia following a CVA) may need to cease driving altogether unless they meet the recommended national guidelines (a field of at least 120° on the horizontal).

- **Dementia.** People with poor short-term memory, lack of insight and poor judgement should not drive. In early dementia, a 1-year licence may be issued, but this needs to be reviewed annually.

- **Psychiatric illness.** Patients with acute psychosis must not drive until they have been well for at least 3 months, are compliant with their medication and do not have serious side-effects from it. The same applies to schizophrenic patients and patients with mania.

- **Disabled drivers.** Modified vehicles (eg with infrared controls and joysticks) are now available; there are ten driving assessment centres in the UK that can assess the patient and advise them on how to modify their car. If the patient needs such a vehicle, the DVLA should be informed. They will be sent a questionnaire, and their driving licence will be altered to show the modifications.

FITNESS TO FLY

The cabin pressure on most aircrafts is equivalent to an altitude of 7500 feet (2286 m). The barometric pressure is around 80% that of sea level, so trapped air will expand by about 120–130%. There are two groups of patients who may not be fit to fly: those who would be affected by a lowering of pressure and those who are not likely to tolerate even mild additional hypoxia. Patients must also have a minimum level of mobility and be able to sit upright in an aeroplane seat during takeoff and landing. Pregnant women are usually allowed to fly until the end of the 35th week of pregnancy for international flights and the 36th week for domestic flights. Babies can fly after they are more than two days old. The airline will make the final decision about any medical condition.

HYPOBARIC CONDITIONS: CONTRAINDICATIONS

- Recent craniotomy or air encephalogram
- Recent chest, middle ear or abdominal surgery (within 10 days)
- Recent gastrointestinal (GI) bleed
- Pneumothorax without a chest drain occurring within 14 days of the flight
- Acute otitis media
- Acute bowel obstruction
- Sinus haemorrhage
- Penetrating eye injury
- Deep sea diving less than 48 hours before flying; this can produce the 'bends'
- Patients who have just been fitted with a plaster cast (within 24 hours for short-haul flights and 48 hours for a long-haul flight).

HYPOXIC CONDITIONS: CONTRAINDICATIONS

- Within 7–10 days of an acute MI for short-haul flights and 14 days for long-haul flights
- Within 3 days of acute CVA

- Patients with uncontrolled cardiac failure within the past 3 weeks; even compensated cases of cardiac failure may decompensate at altitude

- Patients needing supplementary oxygen at sea level should be weaned off it before air travel; these patients will need to travel with supplementary oxygen (enough to provide a flow of 2 l/min) and may need to be accompanied by a medical professional

- Patients who cannot walk for more than 50 metres on the flat without oxygen (although flying may be possible with supplementary oxygen)

- Severely anaemic patients (Hb <7.5 g/dl), particularly if of acute onset

- Patients with sickle cell disease may have a crisis.

CHAPTER 4
ENDOCRINOLOGY

CHAPTER 4
ENDOCRINOLOGY

DIABETES MELLITUS

The World Health Organisation (WHO) definition of diabetes mellitus is as follows:

- Fasting plasma glucose ≥7 mmol/l (fasting is defined as no calorie intake for at least 8 hours) or whole blood (ie done by a finger-prick sample) ≥ 6.1 mmol/l

- Random plasma glucose ≥11.1 mmol/l

- Two-hour plasma glucose ≥ 11.1 mmol/l during an oral glucose tolerance test using a 75-g glucose load.

This applies only if the patient is symptomatic (ie has symptoms of polyuria, polydipsia and unexplained weight loss). If there are no symptoms, the diagnosis should be confirmed by a repeat test. If the fasting or random glucose is not diagnostic, a glucose tolerance test should be done.

Impaired fasting glucose is defined as a fasting plasma glucose of between 6.1 mmol/l and 7 mmol/l.

Impaired glucose tolerance is defined as a 2-hour plasma glucose of between 7.8 mmol/l and 11.1 mmol/l after a 75-g glucose load, with a fasting plasma glucose <7 mmol/l. About 50% of patients with impaired glucose tolerance will develop diabetes over 10 years, 25% will revert back to normal and 25% will have persistent impaired glucose tolerance. Exercise (150 minutes per week) and a low-calorie diet can help to prevent progression to diabetes (NEJM 2002; 346: 393–401).

There is mounting evidence that impaired glucose tolerance and impaired fasting glucose are also risk factors for CVD. One observational study of more than 10 000 patients based in Norfolk found a significant relationship between all-cause mortality, CVD and glycosylated haemoglobin (HbA1c), even in non-diabetic people (*Annals of Internal Medicine* 2004; **141**: 413–430). An HbA1c of >5.5% is abnormal.

TARGETS FOR GLYCAEMIC CONTROL (NICE 2002)

HbA1c should be measured every 2–6 months, depending on how well the patient is controlled and whether there has been any change made to their medication. An HbA1c of <6.5% is considered to be indicative of 'good control' and between 6.5% and 7.5% is 'moderate'. Patients at high risk of macrovascular complications should aim for the lower target, but elderly patients who are at risk of iatrogenic hypoglycaemia can be maintained at the higher end of the range. In frail older patients with multiple co-morbidities, it is reasonable to simply reduce blood sugars to a level at which the patient no longer suffers from glycosuria, polyuria, polydipsia or continuing weight loss; in this case, monitoring may be done by testing the urine alone. Glycosuria can be a particular problem in elderly diabetics and often leads to urinary tract infection.

Note that HbA1c measurements cannot be used in patients with haemoglobinopathies; for example, people with sickle cell anaemia will have artificially low readings.

MICROALBUMINURIA

This is defined as a urinary albumin:creatinine ratio >2.5 mg/mmol in men or >3.5 mg/mmol in women (usually tested on an early morning urine sample by a dipstick test).

Proteinuria is defined as a urinary albumin excretion rate of >300 mg/24 h or urinary protein excretion >500 mg/24 h.

ACE inhibitors and ARBs reduce microalbuminuria and delay the onset of established proteinuria, although some trials have found that ACE inhibitors alone reduce all-cause mortality (*British Medical Journal* 2004; **329**: 828–31). If possible, these drugs should always be used for patients with evidence of diabetic nephropathy; without treatment, the annual rate of progression from microalbuminuria to proteinuria is about 2.8%. Blood pressure should be kept to the lowest level that the patient can tolerate (<130/80 mmHg). Patients with nephropathy have a much higher incidence of CVD, and so other risk factors such as hyperlipidaemia should be well controlled.

Examples of doses of ACE inhibitors and ARBs that are usually required for patients with microalbuminuria are:

- Enalapril 10 mg bd
- Lisinopril 20 mg od
- Ramipril 2.5 mg od
- Losartan 50 mg od.

Low dose ACE inhibitor treatment in microalbuminuria is unlikely to alter outcomes (DIABHYCARtrial; *BMJ* 2004; 328: 495–8)

Diabetic patients who have a serum creatinine of >150 μmol/l (or 130 μmol/l in women) and those with fixed proteinuria should probably be referred to a renal unit.

INTERCURRENT ILLNESS

Type 1 diabetics should always be advised to continue their insulin during any intercurrent illness such as gastroenteritis. However, if a type 2 diabetic is suffering from diarrhoea or vomiting, they may need to temporarily stop using insulin.

DIABETES MELLITUS AND THE GMS CONTRACT

In order to be awarded maximum quality points, practices must achieve the following standards, which apply to both type 1 and type 2 diabetics:

- There should be a diabetic register in place.

- A BMI should have been recorded for 90% of patients within the past 15 months.

- 90% of patients should have had their smoking status recorded within the past 15 months (except patients who have never smoked) and have been given smoking cessation advice if appropriate.

- 90% should have had a record of their HbA1c within the past 15 months: 50% of patients should have a level of ≤7.4% and 85% should have a level of ≤10%.

- 90% should have had retinal screening within the past 15 months.

- 90% should have had a foot examination (including assessment of neuropathy and a peripheral pulse check).

- 90% should have had a record of BP within the past 15 months. 55% should have a BP of ≤145/85 mmHg.

- 90% should have had a creatinine test and a microalbuminuria test within the past 15 months. 70% of patients who test positive for micro-albuminuria or proteinuria should be on an ACE inhibitor or an ARB.

- 90% should have had a record of their total cholesterol within the past 15 months. 60% should have a cholesterol of ≤5 mmol/l.

- 85% should have an annual influenza immunisation.

TREATMENT CHOICES FOR TYPE 2 DIABETES

Metformin

This is usually first choice for most patients with type 2 diabetes, especially if they are obese (BMI >25 kg/m^2 or >23 kg/m^2 in South Asians). Its use has been supported by the UKPDS study (*Lancet* 1998; 352: 854–65) which suggested that metformin might reduce cardiovascular events as well as having effect on blood glucose. It is usually contraindicated if the serum creatinine is >130 μmol/l (although it is sometimes used with caution in patients with a creatinine of up to 170 μmol/l). Metformin should be started at a dose of 500 mg od for 1 week, then increased to twice daily for a week and then gradually titrated up over a few weeks to a maximum of 1 g tds; this is in order to reduce the incidence of gastrointestinal side-effects. Metformin takes several weeks to improve symptoms, whereas sulphonylureas work quickly.

Thiazolidinediones (TZDs)

These drugs are more commonly referred to as the 'glitazones' and they work by enhancing insulin sensitivity. They are indicated in type 2 diabetes as an adjunct to metformin or to a sulphonylurea (if metformin is inappropriate). They should be considered if the combination of metformin and a sulphonylurea or meglitinide analogue cannot be tolerated or if one of these drugs is contraindicated (NICE 2003). Triple therapy with metformin, a sulphonylurea and a glitazone has recently been licensed. Glitazones may take a few weeks to achieve maximum effectiveness, so an initial deterioration in glycaemic control is to be expected if they are changed from another treatment.

Insulin secretagogues

This group includes the sulphonylureas and the meglitinide analogues such as repaglinide. Unless there is a special reason, a sulphonylurea rather than a meglitinide should be used initially. Shorter-acting sulphonylureas, such as tolbutamide, gliclazide or glipizide are less likely to cause hypoglycaemia and can be used in patients with renal impairment. Of the longer-acting agents, glimepiride is less likely than glibenclamide to cause hypoglycaemia.

The meglitinide analogues are short-acting (no more than 3 hours) and take effect within 15 minutes; they are therefore theoretically useful in reducing postprandial hyperglycaemia.

Insulin secretagogues can be used in combination with metformin for people who need better glycaemic control and may sometimes be used as first-line treatment if the patient is not obese or cannot tolerate metformin.

Acarbose

Acarbose can be used in people who are unable to tolerate other classes of oral hypoglycaemics, but often produces unacceptable side-effects of flatulence and bloating. These can be minimised by slow introduction. It has only a modest effect in lowering blood sugar and may be used as an adjunct to other treatments.

CONVERTING TYPE 2 DIABETICS TO INSULIN

Insulin may be required for type 2 diabetics who continue to lose weight or who are symptomatic without it; such people usually feel much better on insulin treatment. It is also helpful when better glycaemic control is desirable. Insulin is not recommended for obese type 2 diabetics who are continuing to put on weight, as the problem will get worse when they start insulin.

Most type 2 diabetics who are being considered for insulin are probably already on maximum doses of oral hypoglycaemics. Insulin can usually be initiated in primary care, if the following points are noted:

- Stop meglitinide analogues and thiazolidinediones; there is a concern that when TZDs are given in combination with insulin, they can exacerbate heart failure by increasing fluid retention. However, this combination is licensed in the USA.

- If the patient is on a combination of metformin and a sulphonylurea, continue the metformin. The clinician can choose whether or not to continue the sulphonylurea.

- If the patient is on a combination of a sulphonylurea with an oral hypoglycaemic other than metformin, continue the sulphonylurea and stop the other agent (NICE 2002). If the patient is not controlled with once-daily isophane insulin (Insulatard®) after 3–6 months, stop the sulphonylurea.

- Metformin is usually continued at the same dose.

CHOICES OF INSULIN REGIME

- A common first choice is a medium-acting isophane insulin at bedtime, eg Insulatard®. This has its peak effect 4–6 hours after administration and stays in the circulation for 12–14 hours. For this reason, some patients suffer from nocturnal hypoglycaemia on it, with rebound hyperglycaemia in the morning. Nocturnal hypoglycaemia should be suspected if the patient reports profuse sweating overnight (and occasionally evidence of a convulsion, eg a bitten tongue).

- It is reasonable to start the Insulatard® at a low dose (eg 10 units) and then it increases gradually, so that target fasting blood glucose levels of 4–6 mmol/l are achieved. Eventually, most type 2 diabetics will need much higher doses, especially if they are obese; in this case, a once-daily Insulatard® regime will probably not be adequate.

- If once-daily Insulatard® is insufficient after 3–6 months and the patient is young and well motivated, a combination of Actrapid® (tds, taken 15–30 minutes before each meal) with Insulatard® may be tried, as this will potentially give better glycaemic control than a once- or twice-daily regime; in this case, the normal daily dose of insulin should be divided by four, and an adjustment made so that slightly more than a-quarter is given before breakfast and less than a-quarter before bedtime. Actrapid(®) starts to work 30 minutes after administration and lasts for 4 hours. Insulin lispro (Humalog®) and insulin aspart (NovoRapid®) are rapidly-acting insulins that can be used instead of Actrapid(®) and can be given immediately before or after a meal; they are sometimes useful for younger patients with erratic eating habits.

- An alternative regime is bd Mixtard® (30/70) at 0.5 U/kg per day initially, with two-thirds taken 30 minutes before breakfast and one-third taken 30 minutes before the evening meal. Most type 2 diabetics eventually need fairly high doses of insulin, usually at least 1.0 U/kg per day.

- Insulin glargine is particularly suitable for frail, elderly patients or for those with a history of hypoglycaemia on other insulin regimes. It has the advantage of only needing to be administered once a day and of being unlikely to cause hypoglycaemia; its onset of action is after about 90 minutes and it works for at least 24 hours. Insulin detemir is similar.

- Glargine can be started off at a dose of 6–10 units at night. Due to its cost, NICE does not recommend glargine as a first-line treatment for type 2 diabetics; it should be reserved for people who experience recurrent episodes of hypoglycaemia with other regimes, for those who would otherwise require twice-daily injections of Insulatard® to maintain glycaemic control and for those who need help with insulin administration.

INSULIN PUMPS

Insulin pumps continuously infuse insulin subcutaneously over a 24-hour period, and patients are able to give themselves preprandial boosts.

Usually 70% of the normal daily insulin is required when converting to a pump. Half of this should be given at the constant, basal pump rate (approximately 1 unit per hour). The other half should be given immediately before each of the three main meals (depending on the amount of carbohydrate in the meal).

Pumps can be prescribed under the NHS (by specialists only) for type 1 diabetics who are not adequately controlled on other regimes and who experience hypoglycaemia at the doses required to maintain good glycaemic control. They are not recommended for type 2 diabetics.

HOME MONITORING

Home testing is certainly advisable for type 1 diabetics, who should ideally check their blood glucose once or twice every day, at different times of day, so that a pattern emerges over the weeks. The situation is less clear-cut for type 2 diabetics who are not on insulin, and depends on individual patient preference. If a patient is keen to self-monitor, they should be advised to check a fasting glucose or postprandial glucose (1–2 hours after their main meal). Fasting glucose should be no greater than 6 mmol/l and a postprandial reading should ideally not exceed 9 mmol/l.

Home testing machines and finger-pricking devices are not available on FP10, although the test strips and lancets are. There are many different types of test strip that are compatible with different machines; there is a comprehensive list in the *British National Formulary*. The type of lancet (A, B or C) prescribed depends on which finger-pricking device the patient has eg type C lancets are compatible with the Softclix® finger-pricking device.

INSULIN ADMINISTRATION

Insulin pens deliver metered doses of insulin from an insulin cartridge and are currently the most popular method of administration. There are pens available for the visually impaired and some pens are preloaded and disposable. All are available on an FP10, as are their accompanying needles (eg NovoFine®, BD Microfine®). Commonly used pens in the UK include:

- NovoPen®; suitable for 3-ml penfill insulin cartridges, eg Actrapid®, NovoRapid®, Insulatard®

- Autopen®; used with Lilly and CP products, eg Humulin S®, Humalog®, Humulin I®

- Innovo®; for use with 3-ml penfill cartridges.

Insulin cartridges usually contain 3 ml of insulin and there are 100 units of insulin per millilitre; for many patients, one cartridge will therefore only last for a week or even less.

Insulin glargine is available on the NHS only as a prefilled disposable injection device, with a range of 2–40 units.

A minority of patients still have reusable plastic syringes and disposable needles, and draw up their insulin from vials.

Insulin is usually injected into the thighs or the abdomen. Patients should be advised to rotate within a site but not between sites for insulin given at a particular time of day (so that absorption remains the same). If patients inject into the same area regularly, unsightly fatty lumps can develop. The skin should be cleaned and held taut, and the needle inserted at 90º.

Initial problems encountered on starting insulin include:

- Blurring of the vision; usually resolves within 2–3 weeks and is due to a change of lens refraction.

- Peripheral oedema; again, usually resolves after a few weeks.

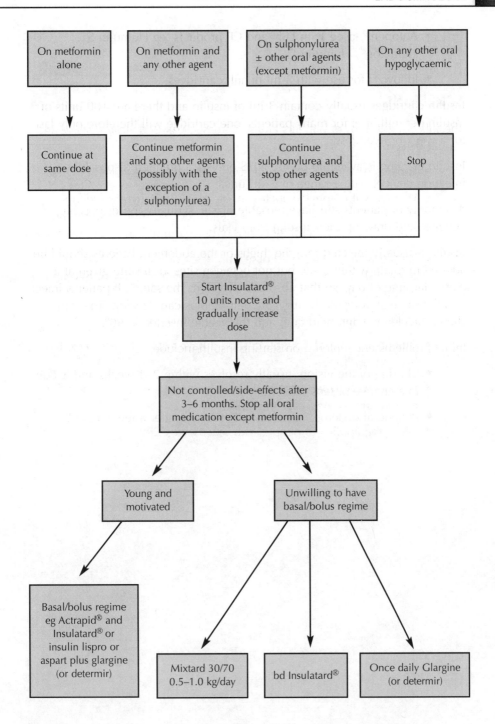

Figure 4.1 Flow diagram for converting patients with type 2 diabetes to insulin

THYROID DISEASE

SCREENING

The following groups of patients are at increased risk of thyroid disease and should be screened:

- Patients on lithium and amiodarone should have 6-monthly TFTs.

- Women with type 1 diabetes should have their thyroid function checked in the first trimester of pregnancy and post-delivery (these women have a much higher risk of postpartum thyroid dysfunction).

- People with Down's syndrome, Turner's syndrome and Addison's disease should have annual checks, as they are at risk of developing hypothyroidism.

- Diabetic patients should also have an annual TFT check.

- Patients with atrial fibrillation should have a one-off test to exclude hyperthyroidism.

- Patients with hyperlipidaemia should also be tested as a one-off, to exclude underlying hypothyroidism.

- The same applies to people with macrocytosis.

HYPOTHYROIDISM

The most common cause of hypothyroidism in the West is Hashimoto's disease, which is autoimmune in nature. These patients almost always test positive for anti-thyroid peroxidase (anti-TPO) and antithyroglobulin antibodies.

STARTING TREATMENT

- Start with thyroxine 100 micrograms per day for young patients or 25–50 micrograms per day for older patients or those with a history of CHD. If treatment is started at the lower dose, it can be increased in increments of 25 micrograms every 4 weeks, according to how the patient feels.

- There is no point in checking TFTs more frequently than once every 6–8 weeks, because this is how long it takes for the thyroid-stimulating hormone (TSH) to change in response to an alteration in dosage.

- Many patients don't feel the benefit of treatment for 3 months after thyroxine is started, and complete recovery can take up to 12 months.

- Most patients require a maintenance thyroxine dose of 100–150 micrograms, although very obese people might need more.

MONITORING TREATMENT

- The aim should be to keep the TSH within the normal range, ideally around 1 mU/l. This usually results in a free T4 in the upper half of the normal range.

- Once the patient is stable, their thyroid function should be checked annually.

TREATMENT-INDUCED TSH SUPPRESSION

Some patients feel very well on a dose of thyroxine that keeps the free T4 and T3 within the normal range, but causes the TSH to become suppressed. Ideally, dose reduction should be attempted, but a proportion of these people will then become symptomatic and may need to stay on the higher dose.

There are potential harmful effects involved in treating patients in this way; there is some evidence that TSH suppression has an adverse effect on bone mass in postmenopausal women (*European Journal of Endocrinology* 1994; **130**: 350–356) and that there is an increased incidence of atrial fibrillation (*New England Journal of Medicine* 1994; **331**: 1249–1252). It is therefore advisable to exclude osteoporosis by ordering a DEXA scan, which may need to be repeated at regular intervals if there is an initial abnormality. Dose reduction will almost certainly become necessary in the presence of a suppressed TSH if:

- the patient develops new-onset atrial fibrillation, angina or heart failure

- the patient develops osteoporosis

- the serum T3 concentration is raised.

SUBCLINICAL HYPOTHYROIDISM

This is when the free T3 and T4 are within the normal range, but the TSH is raised. It is a common condition, affecting about 5–10% of women over the age of 50. Thyroxine treatment should be started under the following circumstances:

- The patient has positive anti-thyroid peroxidase (anti-TPO) antibodies or antithyroglobulin antibodies; the majority of patients with Hashimoto's test positive for these. At least 5% of patients who test positive for TPO antibodies will develop overt hypothyroidism every year, and it is almost inevitable that this will happen eventually.

- The patient has been treated for Graves' disease in the past.

- The patient has another organ-specific autoimmune disease.

- The TSH is >10 mU/l.

If the patient does not fall into any of the above groups, they should simply have TFTs repeated every 6 months; there is very little evidence to suggest that they will benefit from thyroxine, and the risks of osteoporosis and atrial fibrillation from unnecessary treatment should be borne in mind. However, a trial of thyroxine could be considered if the patient is symptomatic, if the TSH is rising, if there is a strong family history of thyroid disease or if the patient has a goitre.

The aim of treatment is to keep the TSH within the normal range.

HYPOTHYROIDISM AND PREGNANCY

Women with hypothyroidism will need to continue their thyroxine during pregnancy, and the dose usually needs to be increased; if the mother is hypothyroid, there is a risk that the fetus will be affected, and there may be a negative impact on subsequent cognitive function. TFTs should be checked at least once every trimester.

Postpartum thyroid disease affects 5–7% of previously euthyroid women after delivery, especially women who have a positive family history or who have other autoimmune disease. There can often be a mixed picture, with an initial period of hyperthyroidism in the first 3 months postpartum, followed by hypothyroidism which occurs within 6 months of delivery. The reverse can also occur, or the patient can be purely hypo- or hyperthyroid. Many cases resolve spontaneously, or patients may only need thyroxine for a short time.

HYPOTHYROIDISM AND THE GMS CONTRACT

In order to be awarded maximum quality points, practices must achieve the following standards:

- There should be a register of patients with hypothyroidism.

- 90% of these patients should have had TFTs done within the past 15 months.

HYPERTHYROIDISM

CAUSES

- **Graves' disease**: this is an autoimmune condition that is ten times more common in women than men and usually presents between the ages of 40 and 60. It has a lower incidence in the Black population. Almost all patients will have TSH-receptor antibodies (which stimulate the receptor) and 70–80% will be positive for anti-TPO antibodies. Around 90% of patients have a firm, diffuse goitre, 50% have symptoms of eye disease, eg grittiness, discomfort or eyelid retraction.

- **Toxic multinodular goitre**.

- **Toxic adenoma**.

- **Thyroiditis**: subacute thyroiditis can present in a painful form, in which case it is probably viral in origin. It can also present in a painless way, especially in the postpartum period. It is usually self-limiting.

- **Pituitary** (eg a TSH-producing adenoma).

Hyperthyroidism should almost always be referred to a secondary care facility to initiate treatment, as management options might include radioiodine treatment. Initial GP investigations might include TSH-receptor antibodies and ultrasound.

SUBCLINICAL HYPERTHYROIDISM

This is when the TSH is suppressed, but the free T3 and T4 levels are within the normal range. It is a common clinical finding; approximately 1% of the population has an undetectable TSH level. The most common endogenous causes (as opposed to an exogenous cause, ie treatment with levothyroxine) are nodular thyroid disease and Graves' disease.

There is a small amount of evidence to suggest that patients with subclinical hyperthyroidism may be at increased risk of atrial fibrillation and osteoporosis. However, treatment is not routinely recommended for patients who do not have nodular thyroid disease or any complications from hyperthyroidism; instead, thyroid function is regularly monitored, usually every 6 months. The situation may be different for patients with established osteoporosis or atrial fibrillation – in this case treatment with ^{131}I may be considered.

HYPONATRAEMIAMIA

Common causes of a low sodium are listed below:

- Drug-induced, in particular thiazide diuretics (especially combinations such as co-amilozide)
- Excess water intake (or fluid retention in cardiac failure or liver cirrhosis)
- Syndrome of inappropriate antidiuretic hormone secretion (SIADH), in which there is reduced renal excretion of water
- Pseudohyponatraemia (if lipid levels are elevated or if there is a paraprotein)
- Pneumonia in the elderly.

INVESTIGATIONS

Measure plasma and urine osmolality (samples should be taken at approximately the same time) and urinary sodium.

- Suspect SIADH if urine osmolality is >100 mosmol/kg, plasma osmolality is <270 mosmol/kg and urinary sodium is >20 mmol/l, especially if the patient is not dehydrated or on diuretics.
- If the urinary sodium is >20 mmol/l but the plasma and urine osmolalities are normal, there may be renal sodium loss, eg in analgesic nephropathy and polycystic kidney disease.
- If the urine sodium is <20 mmol/l and the serum osmolality is reduced, consider excess water intake.

MANAGEMENT

In general, most patients are able to tolerate a sodium of ≥128 mmol/l. Below 115 mmol/l, there is a significant risk of neurological complications, including seizures and coma. A rapid fall is especially dangerous.

- Refer SIADH.
- Patients with a sodium of >130 mmol/l who are asymptomatic and who have no evidence of SIADH, renal, liver or cardiac disease could just be monitored (at least every 6 months). If there is an unexplained, persistent hyponatraemia of <130 mmol/l, the patient should probably be referred.

- Modify medication if possible. If the hyponatraemia is not less than 128 mmol/l and the patient is otherwise well, thiazides could be continued, as long as the sodium is monitored at least twice per year. The patient should be encouraged to report any symptoms of drowsiness or confusion.

- If the patient is ingesting excess water, they should be advised to restrict their fluids to no more than 1000 ml per 24 hours. Occasionally, patients have salt deficiency and need to increase their dietary salt intake.

CHAPTER 5

ENT

CHAPTER 5

ENT

INTRODUCTION

As with everything in medicine, history is important. The list of symptoms below, taken from the Department of Health (DoH) website, should always raise the suspicion of malignancy. These patients require urgent referral within 2 weeks, particularly if they are elderly, smokers, or if they drink excessive alcohol:

- >6-week history of hoarseness

- >3-week history of dysphagia

- Unilateral nasal obstruction, particularly when associated with purulent discharge

- >3-week history of an unresolving neck lump.

EARS

When examining the eardrum, splint the auroscope with the little finger against the patient's cheek so that if they turn (common in children!) the auroscope turns with them, thus preventing ear damage.

HEARING

A crude assessment of hearing can be obtained by performing a free field audiogram ('whispered voice test'). To do this, sit facing the patient's ear that you would like to test, at a distance of about 60 cm from their ear. Ensure that the patient cannot see your lips. Extend one arm and, reaching behind the patient's head, rub the opposite tragus in order to mask that ear. Ask the patient to repeat whispered two-digit numbers. If they can do this, then they do not have a hearing loss of greater than 30 decibels (dB HL). Being able to hear only a normal speaking voice equates to 30–60 dB HL and patients who can only hear shouting have a deficit of 60–90 dB HL. The whispered voice test is a fairly crude assessment of hearing and may miss pathology.

An asymmetric hearing loss is defined as a loss of greater than 15 dB at three or more frequencies on the audiogram in only one ear.

EAR WAX

Ear wax is a natural phenomenon. Wax is a mixture of dead epithelial cells and secretions produced by glands in the external auditory meatus, in order to protect the delicate epithelium which lies therein. The wax is then carried to the outside by the natural process of epithelial migration.

Cotton buds (which now carry a warning: 'not for use inside the ear'!) only serve to damage the epithelium and impact the wax. Hair clips and car keys are even worse, risking perforation of the tympanic membrane. The best treatment for ear wax is a few drops of olive oil daily into the affected ear(s) for a week.

OTITIS EXTERNA

Otitis externa (OE) is probably the commonest cause of otalgia. It is most commonly caused by the trauma of poking things into the ear and this should be advised against. OE can also arise as a result of excess moisture after swimming or a trip to a hotter climate. These patients should be advised to keep their ears dry, either with cotton wool and vaseline for showering or ear moulds for swimming. Narrow ear canals and eczema also predispose to infections. Remember that recurrent infections at any site may be secondary to an underlying immunodeficiency (eg diabetes, HIV).

The best management is to take a swab and start treatment with a 1-week course of topical antibiotics with steroid; systemic antibiotics are never required. *Pseudomonas* infection requires treatment with ciprofloxacin drops and fungal infections require clotrimazole drops. All topical antibiotics carry a warning regarding use in the presence of a tympanic membrane perforation but the risk of ototoxicity from an infection is greater than that from being prescribed a short course of aminoglycoside drops. Failure of the ear to respond after treatment requires urgent referral. Most ENT departments will have a daily clinic for microscopy and suction clearance of infected ears. Untreated infection may spread to the pinna, causing perichondritis.

ACUTE SUPPURATIVE OTITIS MEDIA

Otitis media is a common disease in childhood and is often caused by a bacterium, usually *Streptococcus*. It arrives in the middle ear from the eustachian tube, via a tympanic perforation or via the bloodstream. Patients often complain of a severe earache (sometimes relieved by rupture of the eardrum) and deafness. The best treatment is with analgesics, a short course of antibiotics and nasal decongestants, eg xylometazoline. Deliberate perforation of the tympanic membrane and culture of the middle ear contents is rarely required. Symptoms usually settle within a few days but a residual middle ear effusion may be seen for up to 6 weeks. Recurrent acute suppurative otitis media may be caused by underlying sinus infection, adenoidal enlargement or cleft palate.

The question of whether to use antibiotics routinely for otitis media is fairly contentious. In general, most children under the age of 2 years and other patients with a clearly inflamed tympanic membrane should receive them.

Otitis media can sometimes result in tympanic membrane perforation, which might take up to 3 months to heal (often less than this if the perforation is traumatic). While the eardrum is healing, it should be kept as dry as possible; long-term perforations can result in infections which lead to cochlear damage. A myringoplasty may be necessary for a non-healing perforation.

MASTOIDITIS

Mastoiditis is thankfully extremely rare these days since the advent of antibiotics. It is caused when an untreated otitis media spreads to the antrum and into the mastoid air cells, producing an inflammatory reaction and pus. As a result the patient complains of pain over the mastoid, often associated with discharge from the ear and fever. On examination, the mastoid may be swollen, the pinna pushed downwards and outwards and the mastoid antrum (area under the pinna approximately 1 cm superior and posterior to the ear canal opening) is extremely tender. The patient requires admission to hospital for iv antibiotics and, more rarely, cortical mastoidectomy.

SECRETORY OTITIS MEDIA (GLUE EAR)

This is caused by one or more of the following:

- Upper respiratory tract infections
- Reduced nasopharyngeal dimensions
- Parental smoking
- Allergy.

Most patients present between the ages of 3 and 6 years with intermittent reduced hearing and speech delay, picked up by the parents or a teacher. Examination of the ear reveals a red, grey or yellow eardrum that is retracted or bulging, occasionally with air bubbles visible. Tympanosclerosis is calcium laid down in the eardrum. It commonly occurs after grommet insertion. It is best left alone even though it does cause a mild conductive hearing loss in some people. Attempts to resect it have proved unsuccessful in the past.

The incidence of glue ear follows an exponential decay from 40% of 2-year-olds to 2% of 11-year-olds. At any age, 50% of those affected will be better in 3 months. It is for the remaining few, in whom persistent glue ear could cause educational problems, that grommets are considered.

Ideally, a child who presents with symptoms of glue ear should be referred for an initial audiogram, and then for another 3 months later; surgery may be required if these audiograms both show significant hearing loss.

CHOLESTEATOMA

Cholesteatoma is the abnormal accumulation of keratinised squamous epithelium within the middle ear. It is caused by the congenital persistence of a nidus of ectoderm within the middle ear, or may be secondary to chronic otitis media. Patients often present with a recurrent, offensive-smelling ear discharge and deteriorating hearing on the affected side. If left, the cholesteatoma continues to grow, eroding through any adjacent structures. This can lead to ossicular damage, erosion of the lateral semicircular canal, sigmoid sinus thrombosis, facial nerve damage and even penetration into the middle cranial fossa, abscesses and meningitis. These patients are therefore closely followed up in clinic.

INTERMITTENT EUSTACHIAN TUBE DYSFUNCTION

Patients who present with intermittent symptoms of aural fullness, reduced hearing and a pain radiating down the jaw but who never have any abnormality on examination commonly have eustachian tube dysfunction. This prevents the middle ear pressure from equalising and is essentially a diagnosis of exclusion. Treatment might include:

- reassurance

- Valsalva manoeuvres

- steam inhalation

- a nasal decongestant, eg xylometazoline, for 1 week.

FOREIGN BODIES IN THE EAR

This is a common occurrence in children. Children will often only allow a single attempt at removing them so this is best done in the ENT department. Batteries and organic material need to be removed straight away. Removal of inorganic material can be added to the beginning of the next elective theatre list.

REFERRED PAIN AND TEMPOROMANDIBULAR JOINT (TMJ) DISEASE

The ear is supplied by C2, C3, and the trigeminal, glossopharyngeal and vagus nerves. Any pain from viscera supplied by these same nerve root innervations may be perceived in the ear. The most common are TMJ dysfunction sensed by the trigeminal nerve and tonsillitis sensed by the glossopharyngeal nerve.

The temporomandibular joint is an atypical synovial joint because it contains a fibrocartilage disc. This complex joint can easily become slightly unbalanced, leading to a vicious cycle of grinding (bruxism), pain and further grinding.

Patients present with:

- otalgia

- clicking jaw

- reduced mouth opening

- worn-down teeth.

The best treatment is with non-steroidal anti-inflammatory drugs (NSAIDs) and referral to the dentist for a nocturnal dental splint. Occasionally physiotherapy and even surgery are required.

HEARING AIDS

There are many different types of hearing aids:

- Body-worn aids (still a viable alternative in profoundly deaf patients where feedback is an issue)

- 'Behind-the-ear' (most commonly used)

- 'In-the-ear' (only available on private prescription)

- Bone-conduction aids, which may be implantable (bone-anchored hearing aids BAHA) or worn as an 'Alice band'. These devices are useful in patients with small, absent or chronically infected ear canals.

Most hospitals now offer patients with presbyacusis (old-age hearing loss) digital aids under a direct access system. There are strict criteria so that all asymmetric losses or patients with pain, discharge, dizziness, etc are seen by an ENT surgeon first.

ACOUSTIC NEUROMA

More correctly termed a vestibular Schwannoma, this tumour of the acoustic nerve sheath occurs in only 1 in 100 000 people per year. It is usually a slow-growing tumour which presents with unilateral hearing loss, tinnitus and little else. As such, it is easily confused with the much more common diagnosis of presbyacusis. Any patient presenting with unilateral signs and symptoms should therefore be referred.

NOSE

EPISTAXIS

Nosebleeds are extremely common, especially in children. It is important to look for any cause for the bleeding, such as picking, family history, medical disorders or anticoagulant medication. Usually the bleeding occurs from 'Little's area' at the anterior part of the septum; however, it is important to look for other abnormalities (nasal angiofibromas and hereditary haemorrhagic telangiectasia may present in this way).

In the acute situation, patients should be advised to pinch the soft part of the nose, place an ice pack on their forehead and sit quietly for 20 minutes. If successful they then need to take things easy for the rest of the week, avoiding exercise and hot drinks. If this fails to control the bleeding, they need to go to their local Emergency Department.

Providing that there is no underlying medical complaint, patients need to be counselled about picking, scratching and blowing the nose and advised to use saline douches instead to clear secretions. Epistaxis is very rarely caused by vestibulitis, so it is often the moisturising effect rather than the antibacterial properties of Naseptin® cream (chlorhexidine hydrochloride and neomycin sulphate) which bring about healing. However, Naseptin® is often used and should be applied for 2 weeks. Vaseline is an alternative. Patients with recurrent epistaxis, particularly those previously hospitalised for treatment, will need referral to Outpatients.

RHINOSINUSITIS

Rhinosinusitis is a medical complaint which rarely requires surgical intervention. There are many causes, the commonest of which are allergic and bacterial.

BACTERIAL SINUSITIS

Patients with a bacterial sinusitis usually complain of blocked nose, facial pain, headache, fever and purulent discharge. On examination, the nasal mucosa is inflamed and frank pus may be seen. Treatment is with broad-spectrum antibiotics, a nasal decongestant such as Otrivine® (xylometazoline hydrochloride), and steam inhalations. Recurrent bacterial sinusitis needs referral to exclude any underlying abnormality.

ALLERGIC SINUSITIS

Patients with allergic rhinosinusitis often give a history of atopy, so it is important to ask about pets, seasonal changes, hay fever, etc. Often patients have similar signs to people with bacterial sinusitis, although the discharge is more commonly colourless. The best treatment is a combination of antihistamine tablets and a nasal steroid, often beginning with a strong steroid (eg betamethasone drops) for 2 weeks and then converting to a milder preparation (eg mometasone) once the patient's symptoms are under control. Steroids are most effective and least likely to cause side-effects when taken intermittently. Patients with refractory problems should be referred to a rhinology clinic where endoscopic examination of the nose and allergy tests can be performed.

The long-term safety of nasal steroids is not well established. The possibility of systemic absorption is greater with drops than sprays. Modern preparations such as fluticasone (Flixonase®) and mometasone (Nasonex®) claim no systemic side-effects. Literature on exact course length is scanty. The *British National Formulary* recommends dose reduction once symptoms are under control and a maximum treatment period of 3 months.

ATYPICAL MIGRAINES

Many patients complain of transient facial pains, often associated with nasal stuffiness; yet when the nose is examined, there is no evidence of inflammation or blockage. These patients are often actually suffering from atypical migraines, which improve significantly with appropriate treatment. However, it may be difficult to persuade people that their symptoms do not arise from the nose, particularly if they have had nasal surgery in the past.

FRACTURED NOSE

Having ensured that there is no laceration that needs suturing, exposed bone or septal haematoma, all suspected fractured noses can wait for 5–10 days before referral. This enables the swelling to settle before assessment, while still leaving sufficient time for a manipulation under anaesthetic before the bones fuse.

THROAT

Examination of the vocal cords with mirrors is usually unnecessary in general practice as all patients will undergo flexible nasoendoscopy in the clinic, which is a far more sensitive method of picking up pathology.

TONSILLECTOMY

Indications for tonsillectomy (Table 5.1) can be absolute or relative

Absolute:	Suspected malignancy
	Obstructive sleep apnoea
Relative:	Recurrent acute tonsillitis (defined as more than 5 episodes in a year for more than 2 years). Some hospitals now have a direct referral system, enabling GPs to put patients straight onto the waiting list)
	Repeated quinsy
	Part of a palatoplasty operation for snoring
	Part of the management of guttate psoriasis
	Halitosis

Table 5.1: Indications for tonsillectomy

HOARSENESS

All patients with a >6-week history of hoarseness require referral to an ENT specialist. The main aim is to distinguish possible cancer from less sinister causes.

Laryngeal malignancy is most commonly seen in elderly patients, often men, who have a history of smoking and/or drinking. They often present with a persistent progressive hoarseness, which may be associated with dysphagia, weight loss and cervical lymphadenopathy. Small tumours are often removed with a laser or treated with radiotherapy. Larger tumours may also be amenable to laser but are more commonly treated surgically or with a combination of chemo- and radiotherapy.

Other causes of hoarseness include laryngitis, which may be infective (bacterial, viral), chemical (inhaled irritants, eg smoking) or environmental, eg voice overuse or air conditioning. Benign vocal cord pathology, such as polyps, cysts and papillomas may also cause hoarseness but these usually require a biopsy for confirmation. Functional dysphonia, with or without singers' or screamers' nodules, requires general voice care advice, such as moderation of tea, coffee and spirits, cessation of smoking, and humidification. Referral for speech therapy may be necessary.

DYSPHAGIA

Patients with organic disease usually present with:

- Progressive dysphagia

- Localised odynophagia

- Regurgitation of food

- Weight loss

- Otalgia.

People with these symptoms require referral to the ENT Department for flexible nasoendoscopy and barium swallow.

Patients with inorganic disease, such as globus pharyngeus, more usually complain of a vague 'feeling of something in the throat', which is often relieved during swallowing. Careful history taking may reveal a temporal association with times of stress. Do not forget to ask about organ systems that approximate to the pharynx and thus may have an effect on it. These include postnasal drip, which in turn causes a habitual cough and hence soreness (treated by breaking the habit with regular sips of water) and laryngopharyngeal reflux of acid from the stomach (treated with a proton pump inhibitor (PPI) over a 6-week course).

VERTIGO

History is paramount in the diagnosis of dizziness (Figure 5.1). It is important to distinguish vertigo (the hallucination of movement), which implies a vestibular cause, from a vague history of light-headedness, which is more likely to be psychogenic. The association of vertigo with hearing loss, tinnitus and aural fullness would suggest an inner ear cause. Vertigo with focal neurological dysfunction is more likely to be related to the CNS, eg epilepsy. Loss of consciousness is a worrying feature which merits referral on to a cardiologist or neurologist depending on the history.

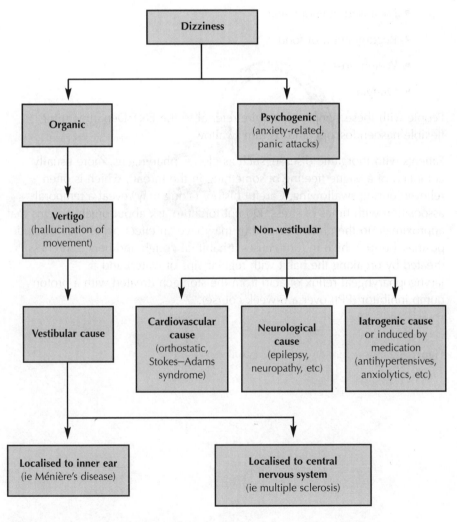

Figure 5.1 Assessment of the dizzy patient

BENIGN PAROXYSMAL POSITIONAL VERTIGO

This is the commonest of all inner ear causes of dizziness. It is due to dislodged otolith crystals (part of the normal anatomy of the inner ear) that become trapped in the posterior semicircular canal (Figure 5.2). Certain movements of the head, such as looking up or lying down, cause these crystals to move within the posterior semicircular canal, stimulating the vestibular organ. Clinically this manifest as short-lived episodes of rotatory vertigo that last only for seconds. Its natural history is one of resolution. Particle repositioning manoeuvres such as the Epley manoeuvre (Figure 5.3) are successful in relieving 80% of patients of their symptoms. GPs can diagnose and treat this common condition.

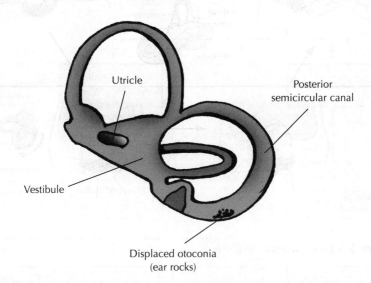

Figure 5.2 Posterior semicircular canal

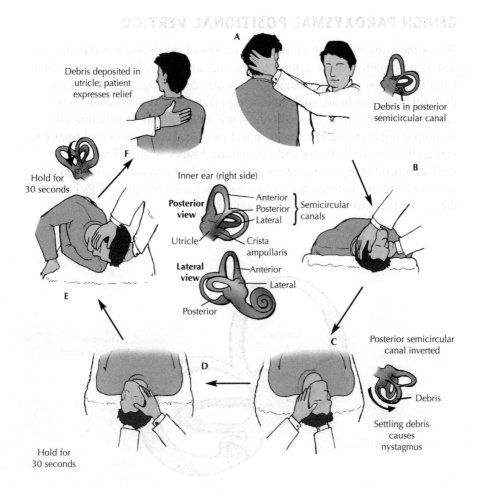

Figure 5.3 Epley manoeuvre

In the modified Epley manoeuvre, the patient's head is systematically rotated so that the loose particles slide out of the posterior semicircular canal and back into the utricle. The first step in the manoeuvre is the Dix–Hallpike test. If the vertigo affects the right ear, the patient is brought to the head-hanging position with the right ear turned downwards (A–C). The physician then moves to the end of the table and rotates the patient's head to the left, with the right ear turned upwards (D). The head is held in that position for 30 seconds. The patient then rolls onto the left side (E). Meanwhile, the examiner rotates the patient's head to the left until the nose points towards the floor. That position is also held for 30 seconds. Finally, the patient is lifted into the sitting postion with the head facing to the left (F).

CHAPTER 6
GASTROENTEROLOGY

CHAPTER 6
GASTROENTEROLOGY

IRRITABLE BOWEL SYNDROME

Ten per cent of the UK population have symptoms of irritable bowel syndrome (IBS), with women being twice as likely to be affected as men. There is an increasing body of evidence to suggest that the underlying problem is one of bowel hypersensitivity to a rise in the intraluminal pressure. Many patients believe that they are allergic to or intolerant of various foodstuffs, but this is not usually the case. There certainly does seem to be a genetic component to IBS and sometimes several family members may be affected.

ROME 2 CRITERIA FOR DIAGNOSIS

Abdominal pain or discomfort for at least 12 weeks in the past year (not necessarily at one time) that has at least two of the following features:

- Relieved by defecation
- Onset accompanied by a change in the frequency of bowel opening
- Onset accompanied by a change in the appearance or consistency of the stool.

Other possible symptoms include tenesmus, straining, abnormal frequency (eg >3x/day or <3x/week), abnormal stool form (eg hard, lumpy, watery), passing mucus per rectum, and bloating.

EXACERBATING/PRECIPITATING FACTORS

- Some patients find that their symptoms get worse with wheat, dairy products, beans, eggs, nuts, alcohol and caffeine. This is not due to food allergy, but rather because these foods are more likely to produce gas, thus causing increased pressure within the bowel and abdominal discomfort.

- There may be associated lactose intolerance. This is especially common in Asians and Africans. Patients with lactose intolerance usually already know that they have the condition and tend to avoid dairy products.

- A minority of patients are intolerant to fructose or to sorbitol and mannitol, which are found in artificial sweeteners.

- Often, psychosocial factors such as depression and anxiety can make symptoms worse, and these problems are more common in IBS sufferers.

- Approximately 25% of patients who become infected with *Campylobacter*, *Shigella* and *Salmonella* report persistent bowel dysfunction.

BILE SALT MALABSORPTION

Ten per cent of patients with diarrhoea-predominant IBS have evidence of bile salt malabsorption; particularly if there are more than three bowel movements per day. It is more common in patients who have had gallbladder surgery or a terminal ileum resection – bile salts are secreted from the liver, stored in the gallbladder and then released during a meal. If the gallbladder is not present or the terminal ileum has been resected, more bile salts than normal enter the colon, resulting in diarrhoea. Bile salt malabsorption responds to colestyramine, but this is usually initiated in secondary care.

ASSESSMENT OF THE PATIENT

Any patient who is over 45 years old who presents with a change in bowel habit should be referred, particularly if the symptoms are of new onset, or if there is a family history of bowel cancer. Diarrhoea is a much more worrying symptom than constipation; constipated patients are statistically not at any increased risk of having bowel cancer. Younger patients with a long history of bowel disturbance who satisfy the criteria for IBS and who do not have any 'alarm features' such as rectal bleeding or weight loss can be treated for IBS. It is worth doing screening blood tests, including full blood count (FBC), iron studies, vitamin B12/folate, erythrocyte sedimentation rate (ESR), thyroid function tests (TFTs), calcium and anti-endomysial antibodies (only in diarrhoea-predominant IBS) to exclude other pathology. Stool may also be sent for culture and to be tested for ova, cysts and parasites; chronic infection with *Giardia* can occasionally mimic IBS symptoms. Main differentials include lactose intolerance, coeliac disease, diverticular disease, iatrogenic gastrointestinal (GI) upset caused by medication, infection and inflammatory bowel disease (IBD).

A food diary is very helpful, where the patient records their food intake, mood and bowel movements for 2 weeks. This often illustrates to the patient that it is not any one particular foodstuff that consistently causes their symptoms.

DIARRHOEA-PREDOMINANT IBS

This is more common in men and it is much more difficult to exclude serious pathology (such as bowel cancer, inflammatory bowel disease or a small-bowel tumour) in these patients; therefore, realistically, most end up being referred.

For patients with a confirmed diagnosis of IBS, loperamide can help, and some patients find it useful to take a dose prior to any potentially stressful event.

Low-dose tricyclic antidepressants (eg amitriptyline 10–25 mg or clomipramine 10 mg) can also be beneficial.

Psychological treatments can help if symptoms are precipitated by stress or if there is a significant degree of anxiety or depression.

CONSTIPATION-PREDOMINANT IBS

It is predominantly women who suffer with this. Increased fibre in the diet (eg 20–30 g per day) only helps people with a previously low-fibre diet; it may make other people worse, so patients should not be advised to increase their fibre intake without an initial dietary assessment. For fibre-deficient patients, Normacol® (containing sterculia, frangula bark) is often better tolerated than natural fibre (and produces less gas than Fybogel® (ispaghula husk)).

If bloating is a particular problem, patients should be advised to avoid food containing fermentable carbohydrates such as beans and cabbage.

Patients who have a normal dietary intake of fibre may need laxatives. In general, stimulant laxatives should be avoided except for short-term use.

Lactulose can lead to bloating; the macrogols (eg Movicol®) are also osmotic laxatives and may be better tolerated.

Antispasmodics are effective in patients whose main complaint is abdominal pain, eg dicyclomine (merbentyl) and hyosine (buscopan).

Psychological treatments can also be helpful in this group of patients.

Fibre-deficient diet	Either increase dietary fibre, or if this is not tolerated, try a bulk laxative (Normacol® or Fybogel®)
Normal diet	Increase fluid intake and possibly exercise. Try an osmotic laxative, probably a macrogol

Table 6.1: Advice for patients with IBS

FOOD ALLERGIES

True IgE-mediated allergy is uncommon in adults, the only notable exception being coeliac disease. Food allergies are more likely to occur in infants during the first year of life (incidence 6–8%), but these children often 'grow out of' their allergy. The following foodstuffs are responsible for more than 90% of acute allergic reactions: eggs, peanuts, milk, soy, tree nuts (eg pecans), shellfish, fish and wheat. True allergic reactions will usually present with a predominantly non-gut manifestation, such as a rash or lip swelling.

Food intolerance is much more common than food allergy and is also much more difficult to define. It is not mediated by immunological mechanisms, unlike food allergy, and patients may present with fairly non-specific symptoms. Examples of food intolerance include:

- **Metabolic reactions**, eg lactose intolerance a patient might complain of bloating, abdominal pain, loud bowel sounds (lasting for more than 2 hours) and diarrhoea, 30 mins to 5 hours after ingestion of dairy products. True lactose intolerance is usually fairly obvious clinically and confirmatory testing is rarely needed. Other intolerances may be to fructose, sorbitol and mannitol.

- **Pharmacological reactions**, eg reacting abnormally to caffeine in tea or to tyramine in cheese.

- **Reactions from toxic contaminants**, eg histamine in scombroid fish poisoning.

- **Psychological or idiopathic reactions**.

Patients who have suspected lactose intolerance should limit their dairy intake to the equivalent of half a pint pint of milk per day. Lactase supplements sometimes help (they can be bought from health food shops). Usually, the diagnosis is clinical, with relief of symptoms when dairy products are eliminated. It can also be diagnosed either by analysing a stool sample for the presence of reducing substances (a Clinitest® tablet is added to two drops of stool and ten drops of water) or by measuring breath hydrogen after a test dose of the suspected sugar.

If a patient suspects that they are 'allergic' to a food, but has not had an anaphylactoid reaction, they should be encouraged to keep a food/symptom diary for at least 2 weeks. After this, the offending food can be eliminated from the patient's diet. Resolution of symptoms supports the diagnosis of intolerance.

If a more definitive diagnosis is required, the patient can be referred for skin-prick testing; this is a very good way of identifying adults with IgE-mediated allergy (but not food intolerance), but is not so accurate in children younger than 2 years. In adults, the negative predictive power is about 95%. It should be noted that, although a negative skin-prick test virtually excludes an IgE-mediated hypersensitivity, a positive result does not necessarily mean that the patient will always react to that food in real life, only that they have the potential to do so. However, if a patient has had a true anaphylactic reaction to a foodstuff ingested in isolation, a positive skin-prick test is then considered to be diagnostic. The patient should be prescribed an EpiPen® (adrenaline) and advised to avoid the allergen in future. In the case of an allergen that is found in many different foods, eg wheat, the patient should be given detailed instructions on dietary modification.

RAST (radioallergosorbent) testing is an alternative to skin-prick testing and may be useful for patients with extensive skin disease or very severe allergy, when skin-prick testing may be hazardous. RAST tests are slightly less sensitive than skin-prick tests.

COELIAC DISEASE

Coeliac disease is more common than was previously realised and patients are now being diagnosed well into adult life. Patients are allergic to gluten, which is found in wheat, rye, barley, and possibly oats. Avoiding these ingredients is very difficult; they are found in a wide variety of foods, including bread, biscuits, cakes, pastries, puddings, cereals, pasta, beer, soups and sauces.

The prevalence in the UK is reported to be between 0.3% and 1%, although there are thought to be many undiagnosed cases. It predominantly affects Caucasians, but South Asians eating a Western diet also have a high incidence of the disease. People with an affected first-degree relative have a 10% chance of developing it themselves.

PRESENTATION AND DIAGNOSIS

Coeliac disease usually presents in infancy (around the age of 9 months), with diarrhoea and failure to thrive on weaning. It can also present in early childhood in a similar way. However, it is becoming increasingly common to diagnose coeliac disease in adulthood, with a peak occurring in the third decade, then smaller peaks in the fifth and sixth decades. The most common symptoms in adults are general malaise, abdominal pain and diarrhoea (or, less commonly, constipation). Another common presentation is iron deficiency in pregnancy.

- 85% have asymptomatic iron or folate deficiency.

- B12 deficiency occurs in about 20% of patients.

- Immunoglobulins should be measured; IgA deficiency is more common in patients with coeliac disease. Patients with IgA deficiency may have a falsely negative endomysial antibody result.

- IgA endomysial antibody and tissue transglutaminase (TTG) antibody are the most sensitive and specific antibody tests for coeliac disease. They are also useful in monitoring the disease, as antibody levels fall if the disease is being correctly treated. Antigliadin antibodies are less sensitive and specific and are rarely used nowadays. Patients with coeliac disease who are on a gluten-free diet may have a negative endomysial antibody test, so if the diagnosis is suspected, the patient should be advised to eat wheat-containing products regularly before their blood test.

- At present, a definitive diagnosis can only be made after taking a small-bowel biopsy; however, things may change in the future, as the antibody tests become more and more accurate.

It is now considered justifiable to screen all adults with presumed diarrhoea-predominant IBS for coeliac disease.

TREATMENT

This is with a strict exclusion diet, ideally supervised by a properly trained dietician. The Coeliac Society compiles a list of foodstuffs known to be gluten-free and membership should be strongly encouraged. Patients are allowed to have no more than one 50-g portion of oats daily; oats are often contaminated with wheat flour. Gluten-free foodstuffs, eg bread and pasta, can be prescribed on an FP10, if marked with ACBS (Advisory Committee on Borderline Substances).

Annual blood tests to check nutritional status are recommended (FBC, iron, folate and B12 levels).

The most common long-term complication of poorly treated coeliac disease is osteoporosis, and a DEXA scan should usually be ordered on diagnosis; if the result is normal and the patient is compliant with treatment, the scan does not necessarily have to be repeated routinely. There is also a small risk of malignancy (eg small-bowel lymphoma, which presents with diarrhoea and weight loss). Coeliac disease has no implications for the patient's long-term health if they remain compliant with a gluten-free diet. Compliance can be monitored by measuring endomysial or TTG antibody levels; if they are significantly raised, the patient is probably not sticking to a gluten-free diet.

INFLAMMATORY BOWEL DISEASE

The peak age of onset for both Crohn's disease and ulcerative colitis (UC) is 20–30 years, with another smaller peak at 60–80 years. The aetiology is not clear, although there is certainly a genetic component. There is a very wide spectrum of disease presentation, ranging from a small amount of bloody diarrhoea or incontinence of mucus, through to abdominal pain and vomiting. Crohn's disease can affect the GI tract anywhere between the mouth and the anus, most commonly in the terminal ileum and/or caecum. Diarrhoea may be less of a problem in patients with Crohn's than with UC. UC can be classified according to how much of the colon is involved (pancolitis versus distal colitis or ulcerative proctitis) and it usually presents with bloody diarrhoea that contains mucus.

MANAGEMENT

Patients should be encouraged to join a support group, eg The National Association for Colitis and Crohn's disease (www.nacc.org.uk). Hospital follow up is especially important for patients with pancolitis, as they have an increased risk of bowel cancer (10–20% after 15–20 years). Patients who have had extensive colitis for 10 years should have 2-yearly colonoscopies. For further details, a useful reference is 'Guidelines for the management of inflammatory bowel disease in adults' (*Gut* 2004; **53** Supplement V: v1–v16).

INDUCING REMISSION

Remission can be **induced** with the following groups of drugs:

- **Steroids**: steroids are available orally, as enemas and as suppositories. Intravenous and oral steroids are useful in treating moderate to severe IBD. Topical steroids are beneficial in distal colitis, although they are less effective than topical mesalazine.

  Most patients will respond to a course of oral steroids within 2–3 weeks. The usual reducing regime for prednisolone is as follows: 40 mg for 1 week, 30 mg for 1 week, 20 mg for 4 weeks, then decrease by 5 mg per week. Note that patients taking prednisolone for 3 months or longer may need osteoporosis prophylaxis and should be offered a DEXA scan. Crohn's disease patients are at increased risk of osteoporosis even if they have not had steroids.

- **5-Aminosalicylic acid (5-ASA) agents**: there is less evidence for these drugs than for steroids, particularly in Crohn's disease. However, topical preparations can be especially helpful for UC patients with distal colitis or proctitis. In mild to moderate UC, 2–4 g oral mesalazine can be prescribed, in combination with topical mesalazine 1 g daily if there is active distal disease. Crohn's disease may also respond to high-dose mesalazine. Different formulations of mesalazine are released in different sites in the GI tract, so the choice of agent depends on the site of disease. For example, Pentasa® is released from the duodenum through to the colon, whereas Asacol® is released in conditions where the pH is greater than 7, ie from the distal ileum to the colon. Sulfasalazine is useful for disease confined to the colon, although it has more side-effects than newer 5-ASA agents. Generic substitution is not recommended.

- **Immunomodulatory drugs**: methotrexate, azathioprine and its metabolite 6-mercaptopurine are effective in inducing remission, but may take up to 3 months to work. Therefore, they cannot be used for acute flare-ups. Azathioprine is the most commonly used immunomodulatory drug in IBD. However, it can cause bone marrow suppression and GPs should always warn their patients to seek help as soon as possible if they develop a sore throat or flu-like symptoms. Azathioprine can also cause pancreatitis; it should be stopped immediately if this is suspected. There are increasing numbers of immunomodulatory therapies on the market now (eg tumour necrosis factor inhibitors, such as infliximab) which are often initiated in specialist centres.

MAINTAINING REMISSION

- Once the patient is in remission, oral 5-ASA agents are commonly used to prevent flare-ups; these tend to be especially effective in UC. The usual dose of mesalazine is 1–2 g per day; and its use leads to a four- to five-fold reduction in the relapse rate. Rectal formulations can be used in patients with distal UC, again at a dose of 1 g per day.

- When 5-ASA drugs are not enough to maintain remission, azathioprine or 6-mercaptopurine can be used, usually for 4 years. Methotrexate is also used occasionally.

- In terms of monitoring, patients on 5-ASA drugs (except sulfasalazine itself) only need a twice-yearly U&E check. These drugs are generally used long-term if well tolerated.

- There is no place for long-term steroid use in patients who are in remission.

Drug	Monitoring
Sulfasalazine	FBC fortnightly for the first 3 months, then 3-monthly
	LFTs monthly for the first 3 months, then 3-monthly
	U&Es twice a year
Azathioprine	FBC weekly for the first 4 weeks, then monthly once stable
	LFTs 3–6-monthly

Table 6.2: Monitoring the drugs used in IBD

Stop if:

- White cell count (WCC) $<3.5\times10^9$ cells/l
- Platelets $<150\times10^9$ cells/l
- Aspartate transaminase (AST) and alanine aminotransferase (ALT) >2–$3\times$ upper limit of normal.

If mean cell volume (MCV) >100 fl, check folate and B12 levels.

DYSPEPSIA

Dyspepsia can be defined as recurrent epigastric pain, heartburn, acid regurgitation (± bloating) or nausea/vomiting. In any patient with dyspepsia, lifestyle advice, such as smoking cessation and alcohol reduction is vital. Medication should also be reviewed and the patient should be specifically asked about over-the-counter NSAID or aspirin use. NICE updated their guidelines in 2004, which now state:

- Anyone with any of the following alarm symptoms and signs should be referred immediately, with the aim of being seen within 2 weeks: **chronic gastrointestinal bleeding, progressive, unintentional weight loss, progressive dysphagia, persistent vomiting, iron deficiency anaemia, epigastric mass or suspicious barium meal**.

- Patients over 55 without these alarm features do **not** have to be referred urgently.

A possible treatment algorithm based on NICE guidance is detailed in Figure 6.1. The rationale behind its use is that most patients with uncomplicated peptic ulcer disease, non-ulcer dyspepsia and gastro-oesophageal reflux disease (GORD) will be successfully treated without the need to resort to endoscopy. However, there is still debate about whether to eradicate *Helicobacter pylori* before treating with a month of proton pump inhibitor (PPI) in people with uncomplicated dyspepsia. **Patients who do not respond to treatment should be considered for referral, especially if they are over 55;** the danger of the NICE guidance is that a small percentage of patients with malignancy will be missed. NICE states that patients with uninvestigated reflux symptoms should be treated in the same way as other dyspepsia patients. In practice however, if a patient presents with purely reflux symptoms, their GP needs to consider carefully whether it is worth testing for and treating *H. pylori*; eradication has only been shown to be helpful for patients with peptic ulcer disease (PUD) and possibly non-ulcer dyspepsia. Reflux patients are very unlikely to benefit ('Bristol Helicobacter project' *BMJ* 2004; 328; 1417–20).

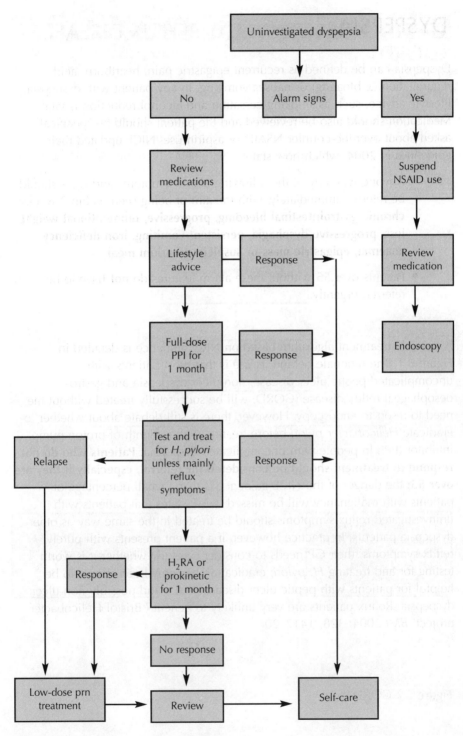

Fig 6.1 Dyspepsia

GASTRO-OESOPHAGEAL REFLUX DISEASE (GORD)

Patients with endoscopically confirmed GORD, without any of the alarm features listed above, should be given 1–2 months of full-dose PPI (eg lansoprazole 30 mg or omeprazole 20 mg), after which they should be reviewed. There is not thought to be any benefit in testing for and treating *H. pylori* in these people.

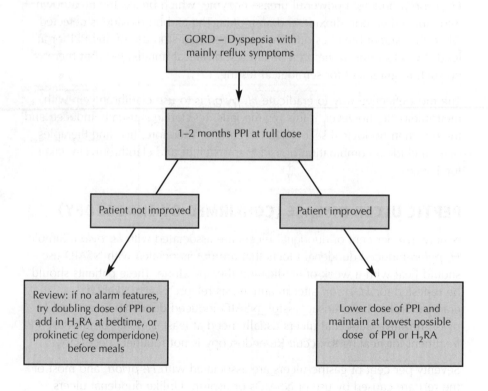

Figure 6.2 GORD

H. PYLORI TESTING AND ERADICATION

Strategies for testing for *H. pylori* in primary care are laboratory-based serological tests (91% sensitive and 90% specific; serology stays positive after successful eradication), ^{13}C-urea breath tests (96% sensitive and specific, regarded as the gold standard) and faecal antigen tests. There are four different ^{13}C-urea breath tests available on an FP10; Diabact UBT® is the cheapest at approximately £12.80. The patient performs the test in the GP surgery, and it is then posted to the laboratory for analysis. The patient must fast for at least 6 hours prior to the test and then drink some orange juice just before it is done, in order to slow gastric emptying (except when using Diabact UBT®, which already contains citric acid in the ^{13}C-urea tablet). They then provide breath samples before and after ingesting the tablet. *H. pylori* produces a powerful urease enzyme, which breaks the urea down into labelled carbon dioxide and ammonia. The carbon dioxide is detected when the patient breathes out. The patient should stop use of any PPI for at least 2 weeks prior to the urea breath test or faecal antigen test, but there is no such requirement for serological testing.

The most effective way to eradicate *H. pylori* is to use clarithromycin with metronidazole; however, if this regime fails, resistance is usually induced and there is then no logical second-line treatment. Therefore, first-line therapies often include a combination of a PPI, amoxicillin and clarithromycin, taken for 1 week.

PEPTIC ULCER DISEASE (CONFIRMED BY ENDOSCOPY)

Ninety-five per cent of duodenal ulcers are associated with *H. pylori*. Simple *H. pylori*-induced duodenal ulcers that are not associated with NSAID use should heal with a week of eradication therapy alone. These patients should be re-tested for *H. pylori* after treatment, as relapse is very likely if eradication has been unsuccessful. NSAID-induced duodenal ulcers and *H. pylori*-negative duodenal ulcers usually need at least 1 month of full-dose PPI treatment for healing to occur. Re-endoscopy is not routinely necessary.

Seventy per cent of gastric ulcers are associated with *H. pylori*, and most of the rest are caused by use of NSAIDs or aspirin. Unlike duodenal ulcers, even gastric ulcers caused by *H. pylori* usually require at least 1 month of full-dose PPI treatment in addition to eradication therapy. Patients with gastric ulcers **should** routinely have a repeat endoscopy, as there is a small risk of cancer.

NSAID USE

Risk factors for developing peptic ulcer disease include:

- Age >65

- Previous history of gastroduodenal ulcer/GI bleeding/perforation

- Serious co-morbidity, especially chronic lung disease

- Use of concomitant medications that might increase the risk of adverse GI events, eg selective serotonin reuptake inhibitors (SSRIs; thought to have a similar adverse GI event rate to NSAIDs – see Chapter 14, Psychiatry)

- Prolonged use of maximum doses of traditional NSAIDs.

Patients who require long-term NSAIDs and who fall into any of the above categories should be given additional preventative therapy, possibly with a PPI, although there is more evidence supporting the use of misoprostol; a recent systematic review concluded that only misoprostol has been definitely shown to reduce the risk of severe GI complications (*British Medical Journal* 2004; **329**: 948–952). However, it is thought that about 30% of people suffer from side-effects such as diarrhoea and flatulence when using it, and it needs to be taken at least twice a day.

H_2-receptor antagonists (H_2RAs) are another option recommended by some primary care organisations; this is difficult to justify, since there is very little evidence that they are effective and they are certainly not as effective as PPIs. Low-dose aspirin is less risky than NSAIDs, but similar precautions should ideally be taken; each case should probably be judged separately.

COX-2 INHIBITORS

The future of cyclooxygenase-2 (COX-2) inhibitors is looking uncertain. Rofecoxib was recently withdrawn due to concerns about its cardiovascular safety when used long-term; it is unclear whether all the COX-2 inhibitors carry the same risk and, until the situation is clarified, these drugs are best avoided in patients with a history of or risk factors for CVD. The US Food and Drug Administration and the National Cancer Institutes recently suspended the 'Adenoma Prevention with Celecoxib (APC)' trial (published online in *NEJM*, February 2005) which was designed to look at the role of celecoxib in colon cancer prevention; patients taking 400 mg of celecoxib twice daily had a 3.4 times greater risk of cardiovascular events and those taking 200 mg bd had a 2.5 times increased risk. At the time of publication, the European Commission was planning a detailed review of the safety of COX-2 inhibitors, to assess whether their excess cardiovascular risk outweighs their benefits in other areas.

Currently, NICE recommends that patients who have rheumatoid arthritis or osteoarthritis and who fall into a high-risk group (see 'NSAID use' above) should be offered a COX-2 inhibitor instead of a traditional NSAID. This does **not** apply to patients who are also on aspirin, as there is then no benefit in giving a COX-2 inhibitor compared with an NSAID in terms of GI complications. An alternative might be to cover the patient with a PPI or equivalent in this case. It is unclear at present whether it is safer to use a COX-2 inhibitor than a traditional NSAID with PPI or misoprostol cover.

Extreme caution should be used when prescribing even a COX-2 inhibitor for patients with a history of PUD; there is an approximately 25% rate of recurrence in these patients.

HEPATITIS C

The Government has recently launched a new initiative to encourage doctors and nurses to identify patients with hepatitis C; it is thought that there may be up to 200 000 people affected in England alone, most of whom will be unaware of their diagnosis. Anywhere between 30% and 80% of intravenous drug users are hepatitis C-positive.

Hepatitis C is transmitted mainly through blood, and the major route of transmission in the UK is through the use of contaminated needles. Screening donor blood for hepatitis C has taken place in the UK since 1991. Mother–baby transmission is uncommon, occurring in no more than 6% of births (although this figure is higher if there is co-infection with HIV). Sexual transmission is also rare; fewer than 5% of long-term partners of affected people will seroconvert.

NATURAL HISTORY

- There is a 'window period' of 3 months (occasionally as long as 6 months) from the time of infection to the appearance of specific hepatitis C antibodies.

- Between 60% and 80% of people who acquire the infection become chronically infected (carriers).

- Between 20% and 40% clear the virus spontaneously and do not become carriers.

- Most carriers remain asymptomatic for many years and have a normal lifespan. Good prognostic factors include being female, abstaining from alcohol and being young when the infection was first acquired.

- Between 5% and 20% of carriers develop cirrhosis, usually at least 20 years after first acquiring the infection. A small minority will get hepatocellular cancer.

The following groups should be offered testing in a primary care setting:

- People who have ever used intravenous drugs

- Anybody who has had a blood transfusion in the UK prior to 1991, or received blood products prior to 1986, or been the recipient of an organ transplant before 1992

- Babies born to affected mothers, and other children in the family

- Regular sexual partners of affected people

- Healthcare workers who have had a needlestick injury (although this would usually be done by an occupational health department)

- People with tattoos or body piercings that may have been done using contaminated needles

- Patients receiving dialysis

- Patients with HIV.

Patients who have received blood transfusions or have had surgery in the developing world may also be at risk.

TESTING

This is usually done with a blood test that detects specific hepatitis C antibodies. Hepatitis C antibodies will be present in anyone who has ever been infected, even in people who spontaneously cleared the virus after acute infection, and so a positive test cannot confirm whether the patient is currently a carrier or not.

A positive antibody test should be repeated to confirm the result. Testing should be done no earlier than 3 months after the possible exposure, because of the window period. Immunodeficient patients, eg those with HIV, may not test positive, despite being infected.

If the antibody test is positive on two occasions, the next step is to perform a hepatitis C RNA detection test (usually a polymerase chain reaction (PCR) test, taken in an EDTA tube), to see whether there is circulating virus present. If a patient is to be offered treatment further tests can be done to assess viral load and viral genotype.

Patients who test positive for hepatitis C antibody should usually be referred for specialist care. The RNA detection test is sometimes done in a primary care setting. If it comes back as positive, the patient should be advised to reduce or stop alcohol consumption, to avoid sharing razors or toothbrushes, to consider using condoms, and to advise family members to be tested (as appropriate). The importance of not sharing needles should be impressed upon drug users. If the RNA test is negative, it should be repeated in 6 months to confirm viral clearance.

TREATMENT

Giving subcutaneous pegylated interferon and oral ribavirin for 6–12 months is the treatment of choice. This medication is only given to patients with moderate to severe hepatitis C, who have evidence of significant fibrosis or inflammation on liver biopsy. Patients with mild liver disease are usually just monitored; the rationale for this is that treatment is likely to cause unpleasant side-effects, is very expensive and may not be necessary. The response rate is between 45% and 80%, depending on the viral genotype and the presence of co-morbidities. Treatment is contraindicated in pregnancy, but can sometimes be given to injecting drug users and ex-alcoholics. Alcohol abuse reduces the response to treatment, so there is no point in initiating it in these patients.

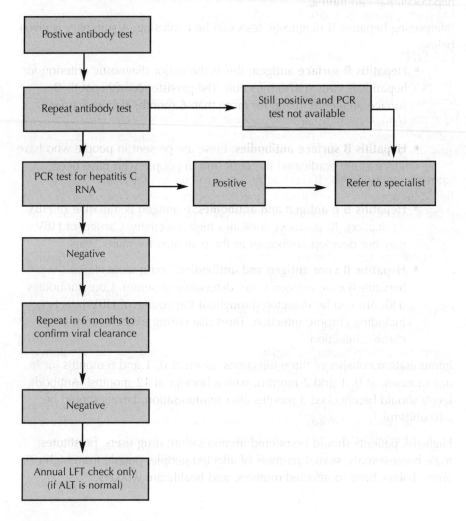

Figure 6.3 Hepatitis C

HEPATITIS B

Hepatitis B is a huge problem in the developing world, where vertical transmission is common. In the West, transmission usually occurs via contaminated needles, unprotected sexual intercourse and dialysis.

The chances of becoming a chronic carrier are high if infection was acquired perinatally by vertical transmission, but low if infection was acquired as an adult; this is why hepatitis B is such a problem in areas where vertical transmission rates are high. Conversely, Westerners who acquire the infection as adults have an excellent prognosis, with a very low risk of cirrhosis or hepatocellular carcinoma.

Interpreting hepatitis B diagnostic tests can be confusing. A summary is given below:

- **Hepatitis B surface antigen**: this is the major diagnostic criterion for hepatitis B virus (HBV) infection. The persistence of hepatitis B surface antigen (HBsAg) for more than 6 months defines carrier status.

- **Hepatitis B surface antibodies**: these are present in people who have successfully eradicated the virus and in people who have been vaccinated.

- **Hepatitis B e antigen and antibodies**: e antigen is a marker of HBV replication. Its presence indicates high infectivity. Carriers of HBV may not develop antibodies to the e antigen for many years.

- **Hepatitis B core antigen and antibodies**: being intracellular, hepatitis B core antigen is not detectable in serum. Core antibodies (HBcAb) can be detected throughout the course of HBV infection, including chronic infection. Titres rise during exacerbations of chronic infection.

Immunisation consists of three injections, given at 0, 1 and 6 months (or in urgent cases, at 0, 1 and 2 months, with a booster at 12 months). Antibody levels should be checked 3 months after immunisation. Levels should be >10 units/ml.

High-risk patients should be offered immunisation: drug users, prostitutes, male homosexuals, sexual partners of affected people, people from high-risk areas, babies born to affected mothers, and healthcare workers.

ABNORMAL LFTS

Mildly raised LFTs are very common and can be difficult to interpret. Because the reference ranges are based on a normal distribution, 2.5% of people will by definition have LFTs above the upper limit of 'normal', with no evidence of disease. The prevalence of liver disease in the UK population is thought to be 2–3%.

RAISED ALT

- Benign, fatty liver is very common, particularly in the obese. The upper reference limit for patients whose waist circumference is >100 cm (or 40 inches) may be 65 U/l. Although fatty liver (also called steatosis) is usually benign, there is a variation called 'non-alcoholic steatohepatitis' (NASH) that sometimes progresses to cirrhosis. Only a liver biopsy can differentiate between the two conditions, but most experts would not routinely recommend this unless the ALT was significantly raised.

- Many drugs can cause raised ALT: antibiotics, statins, NSAIDs and sulphonylureas. Illicit drugs such as Ecstasy can also raise ALT.

- Chronic hepatitis (B and C) can cause mild to moderate (2–5 times the upper limit of normal) rises in ALT; only patients with risk factors need to be screened.

- Alcoholic liver disease: **an AST/ALT ratio >2 is very suggestive of alcoholic liver disease**.

- Other causes of raised ALT are: autoimmune liver disease, haemochromatosis, Wilson's disease, coeliac disease and alpha$_1$-antitrypsin deficiency.

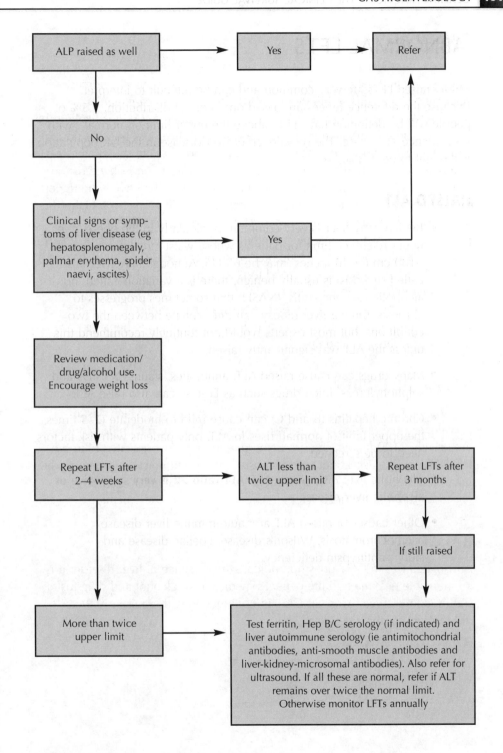

Figure 6.4 Management of raised ALT

RAISED ALP

This can be raised as a result of bone disease (eg in Osteomalacia or Paget's disease) or cholestatic liver disease (eg primary biliary cirrhosis, primary sclerosing cholangitis or biliary tree obstruction). If gamma-glutamyl transferase (GGT) is also raised, the alkaline phosphatase (ALP) is likely to be of hepatic origin, although it may come from both liver and bone. A normal GGT means that the ALP probably comes from bone. Isoenzyme analysis can be done to elucidate the source of the ALP if necessary. An isolated rise in ALP in an elderly person may not be significant if less than twice the upper limit of normal; a 65-year-old woman might have ALP levels 50% higher than a 30-year-old. Hence, a mildly raised ALP is more concerning in a younger person. Patients who have a persistently raised ALP of hepatic origin should have a liver ultrasound to exclude metastatic liver disease, 'silent' gallstone disease and liver abscess, and blood tests for autoimmune hepatitis. Raised antimitochondrial antibodies are specific for primary biliary cirrhosis. Anti-neutrophil cytoplasm autoantibodies (ANCA) levels are raised in 65–80% of patients with primary sclerosing cholangitis. In autoimmune hepatitis, immunoglobulins are also raised.

RAISED BILIRUBIN

An isolated rise in bilirubin occurs in Gilbert's syndrome, which has a prevalence of about 7%, and is more common in men. Total bilirubin levels are usually <100 µmol/l, the rise being due to high unconjugated bilirubin levels. If doubt exists about the diagnosis, conjugated bilirubin levels can be measured; these will be low in Gilbert's syndrome. Patients with isolated raised bilirubin rarely need referral, as Gilbert's syndrome is benign.

RAISED GGT

An isolated rise in GGT does not indicate the presence of liver disease; it is an inducible enzyme and the patient's medications, alcohol and drug history should be reviewed. A rise in GGT in conjunction with a raised ALP can indicate obstructive liver disease.

INTERPRETING PROTEIN ELECTROPHORESIS AND IMMUNOGLOBULIN RESULTS

Total globulin levels frequently come back as raised, and are now sometimes routinely included in the LFT result; the total globulin level is calculated by subtracting the albumin from the total protein and so refers to all the other serum proteins. If the total globulins are significantly raised, especially in the context of a low albumin, a plasma protein electrophoresis is indicated. A normal electrophoresis scan consists of five distinct zones:

- **Albumin**: reduced in liver disease, malnutrition, malabsorption, nephritic syndrome, burns, malignancy, etc.

- An **alpha$_1$ zone** (comprising alpha$_1$-antitrypsin, thyroxine-binding globulin and HDL). Alpha-$_1$-antitrypsin deficiency causes emphysema and liver cirrhosis.

- An **alpha$_2$ zone** (comprising alpha$_2$-macroglobulin, caeruloplasmin, VLDL and haptoglobin). **A rise in the alpha$_1$ and alpha$_2$ zones in conjunction with a low albumin might indicate infection, trauma, inflammation, or malignancy**; some of the so-called acute-phase proteins are found within these zones, eg haptoglobin, alpha$_1$-antitrypsin.

- A **beta zone** (comprising transferrin, LDL, fibrinogen and C3/4 complement); the beta zone may be reduced in systemic lupus erythematosus (SLE) and glomerulonephritis. Fibrinogen is another marker of inflammation.

- A **gamma zone** (comprising immunoglobulins, factor VIII, C-reactive protein (CRP) and alpha-fetoprotein). The gamma zone can be diffusely raised by many diseases, including chronic infection, liver cirrhosis, SLE and rheumatoid arthritis (RA). The individual immunoglobulin levels can be determined with the use of protein electrophoresis. Note that an isolated rise in a specific immunoglobulin is not the same thing as a monoclonal band; a monoclonal band indicates the presence of a paraprotein, which is an immunoglobulin produced by a single abnormal clone of plasma cells.

Interpreting the individual immunoglobulin levels on a protein electrophoresis can be difficult. Table 6.3 provides a rough guide.

Immunoglobulin result	Interpretation	Necessary action
Globally raised IgG, IgM and IgA	Probable infection or generalised inflammation	Repeat in 3 months
Raised IgG and IgA with normal IgM	Possible autoimmune hepatitis or sarcoidosis	Take a history and examine the patient looking for signs of liver disease; check that LFTs are normal
Isolated rise in IgG with no monoclonal band	Possible Sjögren's syndrome	If diagnosis clinically likely, confirm with anti-Ro and anti-La antibodies
Isolated rise in IgM with no monoclonal band	Exclude primary biliary cirrhosis	Check LFTs, there might be a raised ALP; raised anti-mitochondrial antibodies
Raised single immunoglobulin with a monoclonal band on electrophoresis, ie a paraprotein is present	Consider myeloma (60% of myeloma cases produce an IgG monoclonal band; 25% produce an IgA band): Waldenström's macroglobulinaemia (an IgM monoclonal band); lymphoma; leukaemia, amyloidosis; and monoclonal gammopathy of unknown significance (MGUS). MGUS affects 3% of people >70. Essentially benign although some patients may eventually develop myeloma	Send urine for Bence Jones protein (free Ig light chains, present in about 60% of myelomas). All patients should be discussed with a haematologist and usually anyone with a paraprotein level >10 g/l needs to be referred
Isolated IgA deficiency	Exclude coeliac disease but selective IgA deficiency common anyway	Screen for coeliac disease
Global deficiency in immunoglobulins	Immunodeficiency or myeloma	Send urine for Bence-Jones protein. Consider within clinical context. Needs referral

Table 6.3: Immunoglobulin level interpretation

LOW B12 AND FOLATE

Patients should be asked details about their diet, even if they are not vegan or vegetarian; they may still have a poor intake of vitamin B12. Excess alcohol can cause low folate and B12 levels and the oral contraceptive is associated with a low B12. Pernicious anaemia is another common cause of low B12. If this is suspected, parietal cell antibodies should be tested; these are present in 95% of cases (compared to intrinsic factor antibodies, which are positive in 50–60% of cases), so a negative result makes pernicious anaemia unlikely. If the B12 levels are very low, B12 injections should be given (six within 2 weeks, then 3-monthly). If levels are borderline and the parietal cell antibodies are negative, the patient could be given a trial of oral B12. Low folate levels should be treated with 5 mg/day of folic acid, for a period of at least 4 months. Referral to exclude malabsorption (eg coeliac disease) should be considered.

CHAPTER 7
GYNAECOLOGY

CHAPTER 7
GYNAECOLOGY

THE MENSTRUAL CYCLE

- The **follicular phase** refers to the first part of the menstrual cycle, when the follicle is maturing. Serum oestradiol levels are initially low, but steadily rise until they induce the luteinising hormone (LH) surge, after which they decrease again as a result of negative feedback.

- The **ovulatory phase** occurs mid-cycle, with ovulation taking place 14 days before the next period. Ovulation is preceded by an LH surge.

- The **luteal phase** refers to the post-ovulatory phase, when the corpus luteum secretes progesterone. **Progesterone levels of >30 nmol/l 1 week before the next period is due** confirm ovulation. Body temperature is raised by 0.25 °C to 0.5 °C in the luteal phase if a woman has ovulated.

INTERMENSTRUAL BLEEDING

CAUSES

- **Structural causes,** eg **cervical ectropion**, **cervical polyp** or **endometrial polyp**. Endometrial polyps can be identified on ultrasound examination. If the woman is >30 or the polyp is causing problematic intermenstrual bleeding, she should be referred for biopsy/excision. Cervical ectropions are always benign and may be associated with the combined oral contraceptive pill (COCP) or pregnancy. Cervical polyps are almost always benign, but ideally should be twisted off and sent for histology (providing the pedicle is not too thick).

- **Normal variation**: mid-cycle bleeding in association with ovulation is not uncommon (due to the mid-cycle drop in oestrogen) and neither is spotting just before the start of menstruation.

- **COCP**. Women on the COCP often get 'breakthrough bleeding'; in this case, if the problem persists for more than two to three cycles, it is helpful to change the pill to one containing a different progesterone (gestodene and desogestrel may be associated with better cycle control) or a higher dose of the same progesterone. Running pill packets together and omitting the pill-free interval may also help. Up to 50% of women on the COCP have ectropions, so exclude this as a possible cause.

- **Polycystic ovarian syndrome (PCOS)**: failure to ovulate results in prolonged endometrial stimulation, with incomplete, irregular and often heavy bleeding; the usual cycle regulator is the progesterone-secreting corpus luteum, which is only formed as a result of ovulation.

- **Endometrial or cervical cancer**: take a smear and refer patients at high risk of endometrial cancer (>40, obese, diabetic, PCOS, other unopposed oestrogen states) for ultrasound ± Pipelle biopsy.

- **Infection**: it is worth taking swabs to exclude sexually transmitted diseases (STDs).

- **In association with the intrauterine device (IUD)**: take swabs for infection and remove the IUD. The Mirena® often produces irregular bleeding; this may settle with time and does not necessarily indicate the presence of infection.

DELAYING A PERIOD

Women getting married or going on holiday often ask if it is possible to delay their period. This can be achieved by giving norethisterone 5 mg tds, starting 3 days before the anticipated onset of menstruation. Bleeding will usually start 2–3 days after stopping the norethisterone.

Bicycling the pill (ie taking two packets back-to-back) can also be tried, but some women may get breakthrough bleeding, especially at first.

STOPPING A HEAVY BLEED

Women with uncontrollable menorrhagia, eg from an endometrial polyp, may respond to high-dose progesterones; for example, norethisterone 10 mg tds for 1 week, decreasing to 10 mg bd for a further week. Once the progesterones are stopped, bleeding will probably occur within 2 or 3 days and may be like a normal period. Tranexamic acid (1 g tds or qds for up to 4 days) ± mefenamic acid is also very effective, and can be better than progesterones at stopping a bleed.

If medical measures fail, the patient may need a dilation and curettage (D&C) under general anaesthetic.

OLIGOMENORRHOEA AND SECONDARY AMENORRHOEA

This means the absence of periods for >6 months in a previously menstruating woman. The cause could be hypothalamic, pituitary or gonadal in origin. Ask about large fluctuations in weight and stress. Hirsutism and acne might suggest PCOS or an androgen-secreting tumour. The following investigations should be considered:

- **FSH and LH**: a high FSH (>30 U/l on two separate occasions) is indicative of menopause or premature ovarian failure. An inverted LH:FSH ratio occurs in PCOS. Low levels of FSH and LH in conjunction with low oestradiol or testosterone might indicate pituitary failure.

- **Prolactin**: a mildly raised prolactin is very common, particularly in women with PCOS. A value of >3000 mU/l is almost always pathological.

- **Oestradiol and testosterone**: oestradiol levels range from as low as 17 pmol/l in the follicular phase to mid-cycle values of 370–1450 pmol/l. Testosterone levels are usually <2.5 nmol/l in women and between 9 and 42 nmol/l in men (testosterone should ideally be measured at 9 am as it displays diurnal variation).

- **Sex hormone-binding globulin (SHBG)**: low levels are found in PCOS. Free testosterone levels tend to be higher if SHBG is low.

- **Thyroid function:** being hypo- or hyperthyroid can cause menstrual irregularity.

- **Pelvic ultrasound**.

POLYCYSTIC OVARIAN SYNDROME (PCOS)

(Royal College of Obstetricians and Gynaecologists Guidelines 33 May 2005)

The appearance on ultrasound of multiple ovarian cysts is very common, occurring in approximately 20% of women and is not significant in the absence of hormonal changes. PCOS is commonly defined as the existence of polycystic ovaries as demonstrated by ultrasound, in combination with irregular or absent periods, obesity and symptoms of raised testosterone levels such as acne and hirsutism. However, the underlying cause is insulin resistance – hyperinsulinaemia in the presence of normoglycaemia. Elevated insulin concentrations stimulate the ovaries to produce more testosterone and reduce SHBG production by the liver.

Oligomenorrhoea is more common than increased frequency of menstruation, but both can occur. Women usually present in their late teens or early 20s with symptoms such as acne, hirsutism and irregular periods.

Typical hormonal changes that occur in PCOS include raised testosterone levels above 2.5 nmol/l (in 30% of affected women), an inverted LH:FSH ratio (a ratio of >3:1 is suggestive of PCOS and occurs in 40% of affected women) and low SHBG.

INVESTIGATIONS

- **Testosterone**: this is often raised, at a level of between 2.6 and 4.8 nmol/l. Levels of >4.8 nmol/l might suggest a different aetiology, such as an androgen-secreting tumour.

- **LH and FSH**: LH is often raised to >10 U/l and FSH is normal. It is better not to test these when a woman is likely to be having her natural LH surge (ie just before ovulation) as figures are then difficult to interpret. It is better to measure them fairly early on in the cycle, eg days 2–5; 50% of women with PCOS have an elevated LH.

- **SHBG**: reduced in 50% of patients to <22 nmol/l (normal range 22–126 nmol/l).

- **17-Hydroxy progesterone**: this should be measured in the follicular phase; a high follicular phase progesterone might indicate congenital adrenal hyperplasia, another cause of virilisation. A day 21 **progesterone level of >30 nmol/l** confirms ovulation in a 28-day cycle (progesterone should be measured 7 days before the anticipated start of the next period).

- **Prolactin and TFTs**: to exclude other causes of irregular periods. Mild hyperprolactinaemia is common in PCOS, but a level of >3000 mU/l suggests a pituitary adenoma.

- **Pelvic ultrasound**: to confirm the presence of polycystic ovaries and to assess for endometrial hyperplasia (endometrial thickness >10 mm).

- **Annual fasting glucose**: particularly if the BMI is >27, or >25 kg/m^2 in South Asian women. If the fasting glucose is abnormal, an oral glucose tolerance test should be carried out.

- **Fasting lipids**: particularly in obese patients. Common abnormalities include elevated triglycerides and LDL.

TREATMENT

- **Weight loss and exercise**: this can improve ovulation rates and reduces the incidence of diabetes and CVD.

- **The COCP**. If a woman is not planning to get pregnant, the COCP is often prescribed, particularly if she has irregular periods. Women who are amenorrhoeic are at risk of endometrial hyperplasia, and should ideally have a withdrawal bleed induced at least once every 3 months. The COCP is a useful treatment in this case. Oestrogenic pills can be effective in treating acne and hirsutism (ie excessive male-pattern hair growth). COCPs that are often used include Dianette® (co-cyprindiol with additional cyproterone acetate at 50–100 mg daily), Yasmin® and Marvelon®. There are advantages in using third-generation COCPs, which tend to be more 'lipid friendly'.

- **Progesterones**: these can be used as an alternative to the COCP in order to induce withdrawal bleeds. Examples are medroxyprogesterone acetate (Provera®) and dydrogesterone, which can be given for 12 days in the second half of the cycle, every 1–3 months. Norethisterone is not such a good choice, as it is androgenic.

- **Metformin**. This decreases insulin resistance and can therefore help other associated PCOS symptoms, including regulation of the menstrual cycle and reduction of hirsutism. Its use can result in improved ovulation rates; it is a helpful treatment for women who are trying to get pregnant and also for obese women or women with impaired glucose tolerance. Metformin is believed to be safe in pregnancy (although there is very little long-term data), and some women carry on taking it until delivery, to reduce the risk of gestational diabetes or impaired glucose tolerance. A more usual strategy, however, is to discontinue the drug on becoming pregnant; in this case, the patient should be counselled about the importance of exercise and a low-sugar diet and will need to be screened for gestational diabetes. The starting dose for metformin is 500 mg od, increasing to twice daily if tolerated, and then eventually building up to doses of up to 1000 mg tds. The patient should take metformin for at least 2 months before deciding that there is no benefit.

- **Clomiphene**. This induces ovulation by acting on the pituitary to cause release of FSH. It is only prescribed in general practice in exceptional circumstances, due to the risk of multiple pregnancy. It is given orally for 5 days, starting on day 2 of the menstrual cycle, at a dose of 50 mg.

- **Surgical treatments**, eg laparoscopic ovarian diathermy.

PROGNOSIS AND COMPLICATIONS

It has been estimated that 10–20% of women with PCOS will develop type 2 diabetes in middle age; this risk is higher in the obese. Overall, 11% of obese women with PCOS have abnormal glucose tolerance (compared with 8% of thin women with PCOS) (*Diabetes Care* 1999: vol 22; 141–6). Lipid levels are more likely to be deranged, with raised triglycerides and LDL and possibly low HDL. Patients are nearly three times more likely to have a stroke or TIA.

Endometrial cancer is also more common in patients with PCOS. Therefore, if a woman is amenorrhoeic, the COCP or repeat courses of progestogens should usually be offered to her in order to induce regular withdrawal bleeds. Intervals of more than 3 months between periods may result in endometrial hyperplasia.

HIRSUTISM

Hirsutism is specifically defined as 'excess hair growth in women as a result of increased androgen production', ie **male-pattern excess hair growth**.

It is important to check whether the excess hair growth is in a typical male pattern or not, ie whether the excess growth is mainly in areas such as the upper lip, chin, chest, back and abdomen. Fine excess hair growth over the whole body, including the whole face, is NOT androgen-dependent and does NOT respond to anti-androgen treatment. Patients like this should be advised to use depilatory treatments such as electrolysis.

Patients with male-pattern excess hair growth or male-pattern balding should be investigated for PCOS as above, and referred on if their testosterone levels are >4.8 nmol/l.

CO-CYPRINDIOL (DIANETTE®)

Dianette® is licensed for treatment of acne that has not responded to oral antibiotics and for hirsutism. It is only licensed as a contraceptive in these circumstances. The Committee on Safety of Medicines (CSM) recommends that Dianette® should be discontinued three to four cycles after the acne/hirsutism has resolved; most women need to stay on it for 1–3 years in total. If the woman still requires contraception, she could be switched to another oestrogen-dominant pill such as Marvelon®. Additional cyproterone is sometimes required in Dianette® users, if they have symptoms of severe androgen excess.

ENDOMETRIOSIS

SYMPTOMS

Endometriosis is found in up to 60% of women who complain of dysmenorrhoea and in 40–50% of women who complain of pelvic pain and dyspareunia. (*Br J Obstet Gynaecol* 1998; 105: 93–9)

DIAGNOSIS

A definitive diagnosis can only be made with the use of laparoscopy.

TREATMENT (RCOG INVESTIGATION AND MANAGEMENT OF ENDOMETRIOSIS (24) JULY 2000)

- **Back-to-back COCP for 6 months** (or 9 months with a 1-week break every 3 months). This is often enough to suppress endometriosis activity, even after treatment finishes.

- **Progesterones**, eg medroxyprogesterone acetate taken at a dose of 10 mg tds for 90 days, starting from day 1 of the cycle. In practice, most women would have too many side-effects from hypo-oestrogenism with such a regime. The Mirena® is generally much better tolerated, although it is not licensed for this use.

- **Other**: usually started by a specialist, eg gonadotrophin-releasing hormone (GnRH) agonists, danazol (rarely) and surgical treatment (reserved for women with severe symptoms, nodules or endometriomas).

CERVICAL SMEARS

Most cases of cervical cancer appear to be related to the human papillomavirus (HPV) virus. It is thought that a woman must have been infected with HPV for about 7 years before it causes an abnormal smear result and 15 years before it causes cancer. The age limits for cervical screening were adjusted accordingly in October 2003, so that women under 25 years of age now do not need to be offered smear tests. All women aged 25–49 should be screened every 3 years and women aged between 50 and 64 should be screened every 5 years. NICE has recommended the implementation of liquid-based cytology, which should reduce the rate of inadequate smears from 10–15% to 1%.

Note that, if taking swabs at the same time as taking a smear with an Ayre's spatula, the swabs should be taken first; otherwise the wood in the spatula can disrupt the cervix, thus invalidating swab results.

CRITERIA FOR REFERRAL FOR COLPOSCOPY

- Three inadequate smears
- Three borderline smears (these women have up to a 30% risk of having high-grade cervical intraepithelial neoplasia (CIN))
- One borderline glandular smear
- Two smears showing mild dyskaryosis
- One smear showing moderate or severe dyskaryosis or any abnormal glandular smear
- Abnormal cervical appearance: common benign causes of abnormal cervical appearance are ectropions (always benign), polyps and nabothian cysts (white/yellow cysts on cervix).

CONTRACEPTION

COMBINED ORAL CONTRACEPTIVE PILL (COCP)

Contraindications

For women less than 35 years old:

- **BP >160/100 mmHg**; if BP >140/90 mmHg, consider other methods first

- **Personal history of venous thromboembolism (VTE)** or family history of VTE in a first-degree relative under the age of 45 (unless the patient has had a normal thrombophilia screen)

- **BMI >39 kg/m^2**

- **History of migraine with aura/focal neurology/severe or frequent episodes**

- **Personal history of CVD/cardiomyopathy or untreated familial hyperlipidaemia**

- **Undiagnosed vaginal bleeding**

- **Pregnancy and breastfeeding**

- **Oestrogen-dependent malignancy, eg some types of breast cancer**

- **Liver and gallbladder disease**

- **Others (including porphyria, SLE, Crohn's disease, sickle cell disease, otosclerosis, renal failure).**

In women under 35, diabetes is not a contraindication to COCP use, although a third-generation COCP is preferable.

For women older than 35 years, all of the above are also contraindications to use, but the criteria for CVD risk are stricter and the COCP should not be prescribed in the following circumstances:

- **BP >140/90 mmHg**

- **BMI >30 kg/m^2**

- **Smoking**

- **CVD risk factors, eg hyperlipidaemia, diabetes.**

Women at low risk can continue taking the COCP until menopause. It may be worth stopping the COCP at the age of 50 and changing to an alternative form of contraception. The advice about the use of the COCP in patients with risk factors for cardiovascular disease may change in the future; research based on data from the Women's Health Initiative Study was presented at the 2004 American Reproductive Society Conference and suggests that the COCP may actually protect against heart disease. As is so often the case, further research is needed to clarify the situation.

Testing hormone levels in women on the COCP

Usual practice is to wait until the woman has been off the COCP for 6 weeks before testing an FSH level. This can then be repeated in a further 1–2 months. The progesterone-only pill (POP) does **not** interfere with hormonal measurements.

Which pill to choose?

Oestrogen-dominant pills include: Marvelon®, Brevinor®, Ovysmen®, Dianette®, Yasmin®. These are good for women who complain of progestogenic side-effects such as acne, vaginal dryness, loss of libido, depression, lassitude and weight gain. They may also be useful for women who complain of migraine in the pill-free interval.

Progestogen-dominant pills include: Loestrin 30®, Eugynon 30®. These are good for women who complain of oestrogenic side-effects such as bloating, water retention, nausea, breast tenderness and PMS (premenstrual syndrome). They may be more likely to induce withdrawal bleeds in women who are amenorrhoeic on the pill, but not necessarily (see below).

Pills associated with good cycle control: Femodene®, Minulet®, Marvelon®, Mercilon®. These are useful in women who have intermenstrual bleeding (IMB) on the pill. **Medically, it is unimportant if women on the pill fail to have a withdrawal bleed in the pill-free week**. A progesterone-dominant pill may be tried, but there are no guarantees of success.

Third-generation pills: Femodene®, Femodette®, Minulet®, Marvelon®, Mercilon®. These are more 'lipid friendly' than second-generation pills, and tend to raise HDL levels. They are associated with a lower incidence of CHD and should be considered in older women, diabetics, and in those with an unfavourable lipid profile. They are good for women who complain of weight gain, acne, hirsutism and depression. In general, they are less androgenic than second-generation pills.

Low oestrogen pills: Mercilon®, Loestrin 20®. These are useful in women who get side-effects with other pills. Mercilon® may give better cycle control than Loestrin 20®.

Triphasic pills do not offer any specific advantage over monophasic pills.

Oestrogenic side-effects: water retention, bloating, breast tenderness, nausea	Use either progesterone-dominant pill, Loestrin 30®, Eugynon 30®, or a low-dose pill or a third-generation pill
Progestogenic side-effects: acne, hirsutism, depression, weight gain, loss of libido, vaginal dryness, or migraine in the pill-free interval	Use oestrogen-dominant pill, eg Marvelon®, Ovysmen®, Yasmin® or third-generation pill
Poor cycle control	Either change to pill with a higher dose of the same progesterone or to a third-generation pill
Adverse lipid profile/older user	Consider third-generation pill, especially low-dose pill, eg Mercilon®

Table 7.1: Prescribing guidance

Deep vein thrombosis (DVT) risk

Most cases of thromboembolic disease in COCP users occur in the first few months after the pill is started. Women who are long-term users are not at very much greater risk than non-users.

	Risk of thromboembolic disease per 100 000 women per year of use
Second-generation pills	15 (with 1 death/400 000 women-years)
Third-generation pills	25–30 (with 1 death/200 000 women-years)
Pregnancy	60 (6 deaths/100 000 women-years)
Non-user	5–11

Table 7.2: Risk of thromboembolic disease

Monitoring BP

BP should be checked before starting the pill, after 3 months (or 1 month if initially borderline), and then twice a year. Once the woman has been stable on the pill for 2 years, she only needs a BP check once a year, unless there are CVD risk factors (eg smoking) or the BP is borderline-high.

Missed pill advice

- **Two or more missed pills within the first 7 days of a new packet** – patient will need emergency contraception if sexual intercourse has occurred. Extra precautions are needed for 7 days.

- **Missed pills between days 7 and 14 of the packet** – patient should take next pill as soon as possible and use extra precautions for 7 days. Emergency contraception may be needed if more than four pills have been omitted.

- **Missed pills between days 14 and 21** – patent should omit pill-free interval and take next packet of pills back-to-back with current packet. Use extra precautions for 7 days. Emergency contraception may be needed if more than four pills have been omitted.

There is a risk of ovulation if the pill-free interval is extended to 9 days or more.

Antibiotics and the pill

The general, advice is to use extra precautions for the duration of treatment and for 7 days afterwards if a patient has been prescribed any broad-spectrum antibiotics. For patients on long-term antibiotics, extra precautions need only be taken for **3 weeks**; after this, bowel flora return to normal.

Evra®

Evra® is a new contraceptive patch containing 20 micrograms of ethinylestradiol and 150 micrograms of norelgestromin. Each patch lasts for 1 week and then needs to be replaced. Women wear the patch for 3 weeks, and then have a 'patch-free' week. Evra® is more expensive than COCPs and should probably be reserved for women who are non-compliant with oral medication.

NuvaRing®

This is a new contraceptive vaginal ring containing 15 micrograms ethinylestradiol and 120 micrograms etonogestrel. Each ring is used for 3 weeks, followed by a 1-week 'ring-free' interval. It should get a UK licence in 2005.

Progesterone-only pill (POP)

In general, unless the POP is started on the first day of the cycle or when a woman is lactating, extra precautions should be used for the first 7 days. It should be taken at the same time every day (there is a 'missed pill window' of 3 hours). Women over 70 kg should consider taking two POPs a day, particularly if they are young (eg < 30). **If the 3-hour window period is missed, extra precautions should be used for 7 days and if sexual intercourse takes place within 48 hours following the delay, emergency contraception will be needed.**

Cerazette® has a higher dose of progesterone than other pills and inhibits ovulation in most women who take it; it is now marketed as having a 12-hour 'missed pill window' period, compared with 3 hours for the other POPs. It is more effective than other POPs and may therefore be better for younger women. There is no need to increase the dose in obese women.

PROGESTERONE INJECTIONS

Depo-Provera® can generally be used for about 5 years at a stretch before alternatives are considered, although the CSM recommends reviewing the patient every 2 years to assess whether the benefits still outweigh the risks. Oestrogen levels should be checked if a woman has been receiving injections for >5 years or if she has symptoms of hypo-oestrogenism, eg dry vagina, low libido, depression, acne, breakthrough bleeding. If oestrogen levels are going to be checked, a blood sample should be taken just before the next injection is due. Oestradiol levels of <100 pmol/l are considered low, and alternative forms of contraception should be discussed. It is worth noting that amenorrhoea alone is **not** a good reason for checking oestradiol levels; this does not automatically indicate hypo-oestrogenism, just as having periods is not a sufficient reassurance. However, women who have been amenorrhoeic for >3 years should be questioned about symptoms of hypo-oestrogenism. The CSM recommends that Depo-Provera® should only be used as a first-line contraceptive in adolescents if other methods are unacceptable.

Contraindications

- Women who are >45

- Women with osteoporosis or strong risk factors for osteoporosis (eg heavy smoking, anorexia, long-term steroid use)

- CVD or strong risk factors for CVD

- History of symptomatic ovarian cysts.

Depo-Provera® is given every 12 weeks. If there is up to a week's delay, the next injection should be given as normal, and the patient advised to use condoms for 7 days. If the delay is >1 week, emergency contraception may be needed. If the delay is >2 weeks, the next injection should not be given until the patient has been abstinent for at least 10 days and a pregnancy test is negative. This does not apply if no sexual intercourse has taken place since the date when the next injection was due.

DIAPHRAGMS

Diaphragms can be inserted at any time prior to sexual intercourse, but must remain in place for at least 6 hours afterwards. Two 10-cm strips of spermicide need to be applied to the side of the diaphragm facing the cervix and will need to be re-applied if the diaphragm is inserted more than 3 hours before intercourse (this can be done by inserting a pessary or inserting cream with the help of an applicator). They should be rinsed with soap and water after use. Diaphragms usually last for about 2 years before they need replacing.

Fitting the diaphragm

Diaphragms come in various sizes, from 55 mm to 100 mm in diameter. Exact fitting is not important, but a diaphragm that is too big will be uncomfortable and one that is too small may not cover the whole cervix or may dislodge. Most women will require a diaphragm with a diameter of between 65 mm and 85 mm and, in general, the largest diaphragm that is comfortable is probably the correct size. Fitting can be done in the following way:

- Do a pelvic examination to exclude uterine or vaginal wall prolapse as these are contraindications to use.

- Measure the distance from the pubis to the posterior fornix. This gives an idea of the size of diaphragm that will be needed.

- Compress the ring of the diaphragm between the finger and thumb (the dome usually points upwards, but this is not important) and insert the diaphragm along the posterior vaginal wall, until it is in the posterior fornix.

- Push the anterior rim up, behind the pubis. The diaphragm should completely cover the cervix and most of the anterior vaginal wall.

Most women insert their diaphragms when squatting or with one foot raised. Technique should be assessed 1 week after the diaphragm is first given to the patient. Diaphragms should not cause discomfort, and if they do the size is probably incorrect. Size should be checked after any significant change in weight (>5 kg) or after a pregnancy.

INTRAUTERINE DEVICES (IUDS)

The usual first choice of IUD is the Copper T 380 'slimline' coil (Cu 380 S). It is extremely effective and can be left in situ for 8–10 years. Any copper device fitted over the age of 40 does not need to be removed until menopause. Women should routinely have a check-up 6 weeks post-insertion and then annually. The best time to insert a coil is between days 4 and 14 of the cycle (and certainly before day 20). Removal is usually arranged when the woman is menstruating, but can be done at any time providing that she starts using an alternative form of contraception at least 7 days prior to removal. This is of course not necessary for a patient who wants to become pregnant.

Women who do conceive while the IUD is in situ should be advised to have it removed, ideally in the first trimester. If the threads are not visible and therefore the IUD cannot be removed, there is an increased risk of second trimester abortion. If the woman goes on to delivery suite with the IUD still in situ, she must warn the midwife to check that it has been expelled with the products of conception. If not, she will need to have a radiograph to identify where it is; it could otherwise cause her ongoing pain and fertility problems.

Lost threads

When IUD threads cannot be seen, pregnancy should always be excluded. The cervical canal can be gently explored using narrow artery forceps. A pelvic ultrasound may be necessary and if the IUD is in the correct position, no action needs to be taken until it is time for the IUD to be changed; this can usually be achieved using an Emmett retriever or a Retrievette (most family planning clinics should have these).

Infection and IUDs

Pre-insertion infection: Ideally, an endocervical swab should be taken and insertion of the IUD delayed until the results are back. If this is not possible, antibiotic prophylaxis should be given at the time of insertion, eg doxycycline 100 mg bd for 7 days. If a woman is in a long-term monogamous relationship, antibiotics can be withheld until the swab results come through. Group B *Streptococcus* is a common finding and does not need to be treated. Women are at greatest risk of infection within the first 20 days after insertion of the coil; it is thought that these patients are carriers of *Chlamydia* anyway and that insertion of an IUD allows the infection to spread from the lower genital tract. Women who have a coil fitted should always be informed of the symptoms of pelvic inflammatory disease (PID).

Post-insertion infection: After 5 years of having an IUD in situ, 20% of patients become colonised by *Actinomyces israeli*, which is usually a gut commensal. The presence of *A. israeli* is often only discovered when a cervical smear report comments on the presence of 'Actinomyces-like organisms' (ALOs). There is a small chance that these women will go on to develop systemic infection, which can be fatal. They should therefore be offered a vaginal examination and the coil removed if there are any symptoms of pelvic tenderness or if a mass is detected. Asymptomatic women can either have the coil removed, or have regular 6-monthly examinations and be given information on symptoms of PID; in practice, many gynaecologists prefer to simply remove the IUD. It would be usual practice to wait for a few months before replacing the coil.

Women who develop vaginal discharge while they have the IUD in situ should have swabs taken and be treated with antibiotics as appropriate (eg doxycycline for possible *Chlamydia* and metronidazole for anaerobic infection). In general, the IUD should be left in situ initially, but be removed if the symptoms do not improve with treatment.

Intrauterine systems (IUS)

The IUS or 'Mirena®' coil releases low-dose levonorgestrel (20 micrograms per day) and can be left in situ for up to 5 years if used as a contraceptive, or longer if used to control symptoms of dysmenorrhoea or menorrhagia. A coil releasing an even lower dose of progestogen may become available in the future (FibroPlant®).

IMPLANTS

Implanon® is inserted subdermally during the first 5 days of the cycle. It should be removed after 3 years.

TERMINATION OF PREGNANCY

MEDICAL METHODS

Mifepristone plus prostaglandin is effective until 24 weeks' gestation, although its use is most commonly restricted to pregnancies of <9 weeks. Mifepristone (200 mg) is given orally, followed 1–3 days later by 800 μg vaginal misoprostol. Further 400 micrograms doses of vaginal misoprostol may be required if abortion has not occurred within 4 hours, especially for second trimester pregnancies.

SURGICAL METHODS

Conventional suction termination should be avoided at gestations below 7 weeks because there is an unacceptably high failure rate. However, it is an appropriate method at gestations of 7–15 weeks. Cervical preparation will be needed for pregnancies of >10 weeks or if the patient is <18 years of age; this is usually achieved with 400 μg vaginal misoprostol given 3 hours before surgery. For gestations above 15 weeks, surgical abortion is done by dilation and evacuation (preceded by cervical preparation).

Most centres offer routine peri-abortion antibiotic prophylaxis, with either 1 g rectal metronidazole plus 7 days of bd doxycycline or metronidazole plus a stat 1-g dose of azithromycin.

PREMENSTRUAL SYNDROME (PMS)

The aetiology of PMS remains unclear, but it appears to be related to cyclical hormonal variation. There are very few licensed therapies for PMS, but the following treatments are worth trying in primary care:

- COCP; this should be taken back to back without a pill free interval if possible. If this is unacceptable, the woman should be advised to bicycle or tricycle packets of pills. Third generation pills or Yasmin are preferable, since they have fewer progestogenic side effects (*J Wom Health Gend Based Med* 2001; 10:561).

- Transdermal oestradiol; continuous 100 μg oestradiol patches with cyclical progestogen for 12 days of each cycle appear to be effective (Br J Obstet Gynaecol 1995; 102: 475–84).

- SSRIs; although not licensed, treatment with an SSRI from day 15 to day 28 of each cycle is effective for some women. Half cycle treatment appears to be at least as good as continuous treatment (*J Clin Psychopharmacol* 1999; 19: 3–8).

- Herbal remedies; eg agnus castus and red clover.

THE MENOPAUSE

DIAGNOSIS

- Twelve months of amenorrhoea in women >50 years.

- Two FSH measurement levels >30 IU/l, in association with vasomotor symptoms. FSH and LH levels stabilise 2–3 years after the menopause, and then start to decline after 5–10 years.

Contraception is recommended until the 'official' diagnosis of menopause, 1 year after the cessation of menstruation in women >50, or 2 years after cessation of menstruation in women <50. However, some women choose to discontinue contraception as soon as their periods stop, if this is in association with vasomotor symptoms and raised FSH.

HORMONE REPLACEMENT THERAPY (HRT)

There are conflicting data on HRT, which makes the decision about whether or not to start it difficult.

In general, HRT is no longer recommended as first choice for osteoporosis prophylaxis in women over the age of 50, due to the various risks associated with its use (see below). However, it can still be useful for treatment of vasomotor symptoms associated with the menopause. It is important to understand that HRT is usually still indicated for women with a premature menopause (below the age of 45) and that the risks of using HRT have not been shown to apply to this age group. A recent consensus statement (December 2004) from the Royal College of Obstetricians and Gynaecologists makes the following recommendations:

- HRT will continue to be prescribed for women with severe menopausal symptoms.

- For women who are not suffering from menopausal symptoms, the risks of taking HRT outweigh the benefits.

- Ultimately, women should have the choice of whether or not to take HRT, provided they understand the risks.

Starting HRT

- In perimenopausal women, it is better to start a cyclical form of HRT; continuous combined HRT (including tibolone) is likely to cause erratic bleeding, which may then lead to unnecessary investigations. Some women eventually become amenorrhoeic, even on cyclical HRT.

- HRT is usually started in the first 5 days of the menstrual cycle if the woman is still menstruating, or at any time if the periods have stopped.

- Older women who have been on cyclical treatment for 2–3 years may be switched to continuous combined HRT if they no longer wish to have periods. Amenorrhoea on continuous HRT is likely to occur in women who have only had light withdrawal bleeds or no bleeding at all while on cyclical treatment. Tibolone is also taken continuously and has the advantage of a slightly better risk profile in terms of breast cancer.

- A small proportion (5–20%) of women will continue to have erratic bleeding on continuous combined therapy and may be better off with cyclical treatment, so that at least their bleeding patterns are predictable.

- Theoretically, older women who have been amenorrhoeic for some time already could be started directly on continuous combined treatment.

- There is no value in measuring hormone levels while a woman is taking HRT (except in women who are using oestradiol implants; in this case, oestradiol levels can be measured just before the next implant is due; the same advice applies as for the COCP (see above).

Stopping HRT

This is best done gradually, to reduce the chances of recurrence of troublesome symptoms such as hot flushes. Patches and tablets can be cut in half and tailed off gradually. Women on cyclical HRT should keep taking their progesterone as usual.

Which preparation to choose?

There is no easy answer to this, as different progesterones suit different women. 'Natural oestrogens' include estradiol, estrone and estriol and are more suitable than synthetic oestrogens (eg ethinylestradiol). Most HRT preparations contain estradiol. The dose of oestrogen required will be higher for a young woman with premature ovarian failure or premature menopause (below the age of 45) than for an older woman.

Women who have had a hysterectomy can be given oestrogen alone, orally, as patches, as a gel or as a nasal spray (Aerodiol®). The nasal spray tends to achieve high concentrations of oestrogen soon after administration, and the levels then drop quite quickly. Women who still have their uterus intact should use a cyclical progesterone as well, for at least 12 days of the cycle (in the latter half, from day 16 to day 28). The Mirena® is sometimes used as an alternative to oral progesterone; it releases sufficient progesterone to prevent endometrial hyperplasia but not enough to cause systemic side-effects. It received a licence for use solely in HRT in 2004. There are also patches available that release progesterone combined with oestrogen (eg Estracombi®, Evorel®, FemSevenconti®).

Topical vaginal oestrogens

There is always a theoretical risk of endometrial hyperplasia and cancer with the use of unopposed oestrogens. The CSM has concluded that the safety of long-term use of topical vaginal oestrogens is not well known. Therefore, the following precautions should be taken:

- Use the lowest effective amount of cream.

- Do not use topical oestrogens for more than 1 year at a time; at this point, the patient should have a break from use, to see whether she still requires treatment.

- Any breakthrough bleeding or spotting needs to be investigated promptly with an ultrasound and Pipelle biopsy.

- Some gynaecologists recommend the use of the 'natural oestrogens' listed above, although there is no proof that these are safer.

Natural alternatives (for vasomotor symptoms)

- **Black cohosh** (8 mg/day): however, there have been some cases of associated hepatotoxicity reported.

- **Red clover** (40–80 mg/day): contains phyto-oestrogens, which have 0.01% of the activity of estradiol.

Other Alternatives

- **Venlafaxine** (37.5mg nocté)

- **Clonidinine** (50–75 µg/bd)

Risks of HRT

There has been much adverse publicity recently about HRT because of the results from two large studies which are detailed below. However, the situation is far from clear-cut; for example, a recent meta-analysis of 30 studies involving more than 26 000 women (*Journal of General Internal Medicine* 2004; **19**: 791–804) showed that in women below the age of 60, using HRT reduces mortality by 40%. Although this benefit was not shown to extend to the over 60s age group, no overall increase in mortality was demonstrated in HRT users (including separate analyses for cardiovascular deaths and cancer-related deaths).

Million women study (*Lancet* 2003; 362: 419–427)

This was an observational study looking at the risk of breast cancer in nearly one million postmenopausal women living in the UK and taking various types of HRT over a 5-year period. Critics have pointed out several flaws in its methodology.

Women's Health Initiative (WHI) Study (*Journal of the American Medical Association* 2002; 288: 321–333)

This examined the risks and benefits of use of a particular type of HRT (containing 0.625 mg conjugated equine oestrogens and 2.5 mg medroxyprogesterone acetate) in 16 500 long-term users, over 5.2 years.

Critics have pointed out that the average age of enrolled women was 63, which is older than the average age of an HRT user in the UK.

Breast cancer: CSM data

- The relative risk (RR) of breast cancer in women on combined HRT (compared to non-users) is approximately 2.00.

- The RR of breast cancer in women on tibolone is 1.45.

- The RR of breast cancer in women on oestrogen alone is 1.30.

- This extra risk of breast cancer becomes evident within 1–2 years of starting treatment.

- The extra risk of breast cancer starts to decline after a woman stops HRT and disappears altogether within 5 years after the HRT has been stopped.

- The extra risk of breast cancer does not apply to women prescribed HRT for premature ovarian failure; it only applies to postmenopausal women over the age of 50.

Disease	Extra number of cases per 1000 women using HRT for 5 years	Extra number of cases per 1000 women using HRT for 10 years
Breast cancer	1.5 extra cases with oestrogen alone (no extra cases found in the WHI)	5 extra cases with oestrogen alone
	6 extra cases with combined HRT	19 extra cases with combined HRT
Endometrial cancer	4 extra cases with oestrogen alone Negligible risk with combined HRT	10 extra cases with oestrogen alone <2 with combined HRT
Ovarian cancer	1 extra case with oestrogen alone Negligible risk with combined HRT	3 extra cases with oestrogen alone Negligible risk with combined HRT
Stroke	1 extra case with oestrogen alone or combined HRT in women under 59 4 extra cases in women aged 60–69	Data not available
Venous thrombo-embolism*	4 extra cases with oestrogen alone or combined HRT in women under 59 9 extra cases in women aged 60–69	Data not available

* The latest findings of the WHI study (*Journal of the American Medical Association* 2004; **292**: 1573–1580) show that there were 167 cases of venous thrombosis in users of combination HRT compared to 76 cases in women on placebo. This is based on figures of >16 000 women enrolled in the study for 5.5 years.

Table 7.3: Summary of risks associated with HRT

Disease	Reduced number of cases per 1000 women using HRT for 5 years	Reduced number of cases per 1000 women using HRT for 10 years
Colorectal cancer	**1** reduced case with use of oestrogen alone or combined HRT in users <59	**2** reduced cases with use of oestrogen alone or combined HRT in users <59
	3 reduced cases in users aged 60–69	**5–6** reduced cases in users aged 60–69
Fractured neck of femur	**1** reduced case with use of oestrogen alone or combined HRT in users <59	1 reduced case with use of oestrogen alone or combined HRT in users <59
	2–3 reduced cases in users aged 60–69	**5** reduced cases in users aged 60–69

Table 7.4: Summary of benefits associated with HRT

INCONTINENCE

Always exclude urinary tract infection (UTI) and ask the patient to reduce their consumption of alcohol, caffeine and cigarettes, all of which can exacerbate the problem.

STRESS INCONTINENCE

The pelvic floor muscles play an important role in maintaining continence and supporting the female genital tract. Pelvic floor exercises can be very effective in helping women with incontinence problems, particularly genuine stress incontinence. Genuine stress incontinence is extremely common, affecting up to 10% of parous women; it occurs as a result of the upper urethra descending through the pelvic floor, so that when intra-abdominal pressure rises (eg when laughing or sneezing), the urethra is no longer compressed by the pelvic floor muscles. There is often an associated cystocoele. Surgical treatment with colposuspension or tension-free vaginal taping (TVT) is usually very effective for isolated genuine stress incontinence, but first the woman should be encouraged to try pelvic floor exercises; when done correctly, these are often sufficient to alleviate symptoms. Another alternative if there is associated utero-vaginal prolapse, especially for elderly or infirm patients, is a ring pessary. This is fitted in the same way as a diaphragm (with the same sizing system) and needs to be replaced every 3–4 months. Women who are still sexually active can remove it prior to intercourse.

Duloxetine is a serotonin and noradrenaline reuptake inhibitor that has recently been licensed for the treatment of moderate to severe stress incontinence. Results so far have been promising.

PELVIC FLOOR EXERCISES

Ask the woman to imagine that she is trying to stop herself from passing urine and to tense the muscles at the front of her vagina. Similarly, she should tense the muscles around her anus, as if she were trying to prevent herself from opening her bowels. She should draw her pelvic floor inwards and upwards (it is important not to tense other parts of the body such as the buttocks, legs or abdomen) for up to 10 seconds at a time, and repeat these contractions several times in a row; this routine should be performed as many times as possible every day.

Vaginal cones are small weights, which are placed in the vagina and held in position by the woman as part of her pelvic exercise routine; she should be asked to hold the cone in place for 15–20 minutes at a time, eg when going out for a walk or doing housework. Cones are available from large pharmacists and cost about £15. They are available in sets of different weight cones; women should start with the lightest and then increase gradually.

URGE INCONTINENCE

Most women with incontinence have a mixed picture of urge and stress incontinence. Urge incontinence is also known as 'detrusor instability'. Anticholinergics (eg oxybutynin, tolterodine) can help with urgency, as can bladder 'retraining'. Pelvic floor exercises are beneficial if there is a mixed picture of urge and stress incontinence, but surgery is rarely helpful. If surgery is being planned for stress incontinence, it is important to first eliminate any element of detrusor instability and so urodynamic testing is essential.

BLADDER TRAINING

The aim is to achieve:

- Voiding intervals of 3–4 hours (no more than six to eight times a day)

- Urine volumes of 300–400 ml

- Dryness.

The woman should be asked to keep a 'voiding diary' for a week before she starts the bladder training, and then at least once a week during the training. She should record:

- when she urinates

- the quantities passed (either by using a measuring jug or counting out how many seconds she urinates for)

- whether there has been any incontinence.

The idea is to gradually increase the intervals between voiding (for example by half an hour a week), thus stretching the bladder and increasing its capacity, so that she is passing larger volumes of urine. For the same reason, the woman should be asked not to restrict the quantity of fluid she drinks to less than about 1.5 litres per day, as many of these patients do; patients who persistently restrict their fluid intake inappropriately may be left with a reduced functional bladder capacity. When she feels the 'urge' to urinate, the patient should contract her pelvic floor muscles until the bladder spasm passes. Strategies that can help to increase bladder capacity include the following:

- Asking the woman to sit down when she gets the urge to urinate
- Drinking a reasonable quantity of fluid (about 1.5 litres per day) while avoiding alcohol and caffeine
- Practising pelvic floor exercises so that she is able to 'hold on' when the urge to pass urine occurs
- Avoiding constipation
- Avoiding going to the toilet 'just in case'.

Bladder training usually has a positive effect by about 4–6 weeks after starting.

PRURITUS VULVAE AND VULVOVAGINITIS

Possible causes include:

- Infection: *Candida*, bacterial vaginosis, *Trichomonas*, pubic lice and threadworms. In prepubertal girls, thrush is quite rare and the most common cause is group A *Streptococcus*

- Skin problems; eg eczema, psoriasis, contact dermatitis, lichen simplex (a localised area of lichenified, excoriated eczema) or lichen planus (presents as purple or white shiny spots)

- Lichen sclerosus and leukoplakia

- Urinary incontinence

- Hypo-oestrogenism in postmenopausal women

- Vulvodynia (a chronic idiopathic pain syndrome)

- Vulvo-vestibulitis (pain around the introitus).

RECURRENT CANDIDIASIS

Recurrent candidiasis is defined as at least four proven attacks within 12 months. There is often associated vulval eczema, or one of the other conditions listed above. *Candida* found incidentally in an asymptomatic woman does not necessarily need to be treated.

- Take vaginal swabs and ask the lab to determine the species and sensitivities of the *Candida*. *Candida albicans* is the most common species, but non-albicans species (eg *Candida glabrata*) do occur in 10% of cases and can be resistant to azole antifungals (such as clotrimazole). They can therefore result in chronic infection. Non-albicans species can be eradicated, but this sometimes requires intensive treatment with antifungals (eg 14 days of nystatin pessaries or two doses of itraconazole in the same day). Nystatin pessaries can stain clothing.

- Exclude diabetes mellitus.

- Exclude the co-existence of another cause of pruritus (as listed above).

TREATMENT AND PROPHYLAXIS

Initial management usually consists of treatment with an azole pessary or oral tablet. Two doses of fluconazole, separated by 3 days may be more effective than a single dose in severe attacks. If a woman is very distressed by her symptoms, prophylactic treatment may be considered (see below), but general advice should always be given first; although candidiasis is not a sexually transmitted infection, sexual intercourse can trigger it and couples should be advised to use a lubricant such as KY jelly®. Avoiding soap and perfumed products and wearing loose, cotton underwear can help, particularly if there is co-existent eczema. It can be helpful to prescribe a soap alternative such as aqueous cream.

If these general measures fail and the woman is still suffering from recurrent thrush, prophylactic medication can be tried. Flare-ups are more common premenstrually and in this case pessaries (either clotrimazole 500 mg or econazole 150 mg) may be prescribed on days 8 and 18 of the cycle. If this does not work, the woman could try weekly pessaries. Oral fluconazole is an alternative, but has more potential side-effects. Another strategy is to take daily itraconazole (100 mg od) for a week before the anticipated onset of menstruation and use a pessary after intercourse. There is limited evidence to suggest that using a POP containing desogestrel may be of benefit, although the COCP may make matters worse.

Prophylactic treatment should be continued for 6 months in the first instance and then stopped, to assess the need for further treatment. Some specialists advise treating the partner, although there is not much evidence behind this.

LICHEN SCLEROSIS

This has the appearance of flat, atrophic, 'paper-thin' lesions. Topical corticosteroids can be helpful; for example, 2 weeks of a high-potency steroid cream used twice a day, followed by 2 weeks of a lower potency cream used once a day. If there is no improvement, the diagnosis should be reconsidered.

VULVODYNIA

Simple analgesia is not usually effective. Low-dose tricyclic antidepressants (eg 10 mg dothiepin or amitriptyline at night) can be helpful.

CHAPTER 8
HAEMATOLOGY

CHAPTER 8
HAEMATOLOGY

ABNORMAL BLOOD RESULTS

- **High haemoglobin (Hb).** By definition, 2.5% of people lie outside the normal reference range. The important things to check are **whether the raised Hb is getting progressively higher, whether the patient is symptomatic (eg headaches, dizziness, tingling, splenomegaly) and whether any of the other full blood count (FBC) parameters are abnormal (eg platelets or white cell count (WCC))**, possibly indicating the onset of myelofibrosis or leukaemia. These patients will almost certainly require urgent referral.

  It is important to check the packed cell volume (PCV) (equivalent to haematocrit). If both Hb and PCV are raised, repeat the FBC in a few weeks when the patient is well hydrated; dehydration can sometimes result in an artificially high Hb. If both are again raised, consider referral. In general, a persistently raised Hb of >16 g/dl or PCV >0.48 in a woman and Hb >17.5 g/dl or PCV >0.51 in a man should certainly precipitate referral. Only blood volume studies can absolutely determine whether there is a true increase in red cell mass; these are only done in a few specialist centres. Polycythaemia is most common in 45–60 year olds. It can be primary (also called polycythaemia rubra vera) or secondary (from anything that results in chronic hypoxia, eg smoking, lung disease, gross obesity, altitude). Treatment of primary polycythaemia may consist of venesection or chemotherapy, the aim being to keep the PCV/haematocrit below 50%. Patients with secondary polycythaemia are never given chemotherapy, and venesection is only done in exceptional cases.

- **Low neutrophils (normal range 2.0 x 10^9–7.5 x 10^9 cells/l).** Certain racial groups, eg black Africans, are more likely to have low neutrophil counts; a count of 1.8×10^9 /l is probably normal in these groups. If the neutropenia is associated with a generalised pancytopenia, immediate referral is mandatory. If there is an isolated neutropenia, it is worth repeating a FBC in 4–6 weeks. If the neutropenia is progressive, again the patient should be referred. It is especially alarming if the patient reports that they have recently become more susceptible to picking up infections (this commonly occurs when the neutrophil count falls below 0.5 x 10^9 /l). It is always worth checking the past notes of patients with isolated neutropenias; sometimes, they have had a low neutrophil count for years, but are perfectly well in themselves, in which case it is very unlikely that there is a sinister underlying cause. Causes for neutropenia include: **viral infections, overwhelming bacterial infection (including military TB), racial variation, drug-induced neutropenia (many drugs have been implicated), autoimmune neutropenia (this is really a diagnosis of exclusion based on the finding of a normal bone marrow), SLE, Felty's syndrome and myelodysplasia**. Any cytopenia can be a first presentation of myelodysplasia in the elderly.

- **Low platelets.** This may either be due to failure of platelet production or to shortened platelet survival. Failure of platelet production can occur because of drugs, alcohol abuse, viral infection, myelodysplasia and other haematological malignancies that result in bone marrow infiltration. Myelodysplasia should be considered if an elderly person has an isolated thrombocytopenia. Shortened platelet survival occurs in idiopathic autoimmune thrombocytopenia (ITP). ITP usually presents with petechiae, bruising and spontaneous bleeding from mucous membranes. There are two forms of ITP: acute and chronic. Acute ITP is most common below the age of 10 years and it is almost always self-limiting, usually within 2–4 weeks. Platelet counts are often <20 x10^9 /l. Steroids and iv immunoglobulin are sometimes used to treat this condition, although more than 80% of patients will recover without treatment. Chronic ITP is most common in the 15- to 50-year-old age group. The platelet count is usually between 20 x 10^9 and 80 x 10^9 /l and the condition is relapsing and remitting, with spontaneous cure being rare. If the platelet count is >30 x 10^9 /l and the patient is asymptomatic, then treatment is not usually necessary. If treatment is required, it is usually with oral prednisolone; if there is poor steroid response, splenectomy is sometimes necessary. Patients with chronic ITP should be referred urgently if they are actively bleeding (at any platelet count) or if the platelet count is below 5×10^9 /l.

- **High platelets.** Thrombocytosis can occur as a result of any physiological stress; for example, trauma, surgery, infection, inflammatory disease (eg rheumatoid arthritis and ulcerative colitis), malignancy and iron deficiency anaemia. It can also be due to myeloproliferative disease such as essential thrombocythaemia, which is more common in the elderly and can present with thrombotic or bleeding complications. In general, early referral should be made if other FBC parameters are also raised, or if the platelet count is $>600 \times 10^9$ /l.

- **Iron deficiency.** Any man or woman over 40 who is found to have iron deficiency anaemia needs to be investigated from a gastroenterological viewpoint, to exclude occult malignancy. Iron supplementation (bd or tds, ideally with vitamin C to increase absorption) should lead to a 1 g/dl rise in Hb per week and should be continued for at least 3 months after the Hb comes back to normal. Ferritin levels of >25 µg/ml in the absence of anaemia are unlikely to explain symptoms of tiredness and do not require treatment. It is worth noting that ferritin itself is an inflammatory marker; iron studies may therefore be easier to interpret than ferritin levels.

- **Raised fibrinogen.** Fibrinogen is an inflammatory marker, a bit like the erythrocyte sedimentation rate (ESR), and can be raised for similar reasons. It can be difficult to interpret.

- **Normocytic anaemia.** The first thing to do is to check the haematinics; if the patient is iron deficient, they may be losing blood slowly and should be investigated from a gastroenterological point of view. If the haematinics are normal, chronic disease (eg renal failure) and haematological malignancy should be excluded, eg myelodysplasia in the elderly.

- **Macrocytosis**: see below. Routine investigations in a patient with macrocytosis should include liver function tests (LFTs), urea and electrolytes (U&Es), thyroid function tests (TFTs), B12, folate and reticulocyte count. When an underlying cause is not obvious, persistant macrocytosis should be referred to the haematologists, to exclude a malignancy such as myelodysplasia.

CAUSES OF MACROCYTOSIS

1 **Low B12 and folate**. Low B12 levels can be caused by pernicious anaemia (atrophic gastritis leading to lack of intrinsic factor), dietary deficiency, diseases of the terminal ileum where B12 is absorbed, and post-gastrectomy. Parietal cell antibodies can be useful in diagnosing pernicious anaemia. B12 is sometimes given orally at doses of 1–2 mg/day if there is a dietary deficiency (unlicensed use), but, if not, should be administered by intramuscular injection (three times a week for the first 2 weeks, then once every 3 months). B12 levels are invariably high in patients receiving injections.

Low folate levels can result from a poor diet (eg in alcoholics), increased need (eg in pregnancy, haemodialysis and haemolytic anaemias) and malabsorption (eg coeliac disease). Iatrogenesis may also be a cause, eg in patients taking folate antagonists such as phenytoin or methotrexate. Folic acid should not be given if there is concurrent vitamin B12 deficiency until the patient has had at least one injection of vitamin B12; otherwise, subacute combined degeneration of the spinal cord can be precipitated or worsened. When treating folate deficiency, folic acid should be given at a dose of 5 mg per day for 4 months

2 **Drugs, including alcohol, azathioprine and AZT**

3 **Hypothyroidism**

4 **Liver disease**

5 **Myelodysplasia**. Myelodysplasia is common in the elderly and has a variable prognosis, with some patients surviving for >15 years without symptoms and some developing acute myelogenous leukaemia (AML). Treatment is usually supportive only, eg with transfusions. There is usually a reduction in at least one cell line, eg anaemia, which is frequently macrocytic

6 **Marrow infiltration**

7 **Haemolysis**

8 **Pregnancy.**

OTHER HAEMATOLOGICAL CONDITIONS

ANTIPHOSPHOLIPID SYNDROME

Antiphospholipid syndrome is defined by the presence of antiphospholipid antibodies – either lupus anticoagulant or anticardiolipin antibodies. If it is an incidental finding and the patient is asymptomatic, treatment is not strictly necessary, although some doctors might consider using 75 mg aspirin daily. If, however, the patient has a history of miscarriage, deep vein thrombosis, pulmonary embolism or transient ischaemic attack, then referral for anticoagulation is appropriate. After the first event, warfarin may not be considered essential for lifelong use, especially if there was a precipitating factor such as pregnancy or immobility. However, after a second event, initiation of long-term anticoagulation is normal.

THALASSAEMIA

A diagnosis of thalassaemia should be strongly suspected if the mean cell volume (MCV) is low, but the patient is not iron-deficient. Alpha-thalassaemia is found mainly in South East Asia and West Africa, the prevalence being 20–30% in these countries. There are four genes coding for alpha-globin per cell, and clinical manifestations depend on how many of these genes are deleted in a particular individual. Deletion of one or two genes does not produce symptoms, although the patient may be slightly anaemic, with a low MCV. Deletion of three genes causes HbH disease, which has a variable presentation; patients are usually anaemic, with haemoglobin concentrations of between 7 and 11 g/dl. Deletion of all four genes is not compatible with life and results in Hb Bart's hydrops fetalis syndrome.

Beta-thalassaemia trait is common in southern Europe, South East Asia, Africa, the Middle East, South Asia and China. Heterozygous beta-thalassaemia does not usually produce symptoms, although patients may be mildly anaemic with a low MCV. Homozygous beta-thalassaemia results in either beta-thalassaemia major (Cooley's disease), which presents with severe anaemia and failure to thrive in infancy, or in beta-thalassaemia intermedia, which results in a moderate anaemia after the age of 1–2 years. Patients with the latter usually remain fairly well and only require transfusions during intercurrent illness.

Beta-thalassaemia trait is excluded by Hb electrophoresis, but alpha-thalassaemia trait is not. If diagnosis of alpha-thalassaemia is required, for example in antenatal screening, this is done with DNA studies.

LYMPH NODES

Refer any adult with a persistent, progressively-growing lymph node of >0.5 cm, even if they are entirely well, probably within 4 weeks. Patients with lymphoma are often systemically well; only a third will be symptomatic at presentation. Other possible causes of persistent nodes include viral infection (especially Epstein–Barr virus (EBV) and cytomegalovirus (CMV)), bacterial infection (eg TB), toxoplasmosis and other neoplasms.

CHAPTER 9
NEUROLOGY

CHAPTER 9
NEUROLOGY

HEADACHES

MIGRAINES

Diagnosis (British Association for the Study of Headache 2004 Guidelines)

The patient must have suffered from at least five episodes of a headache lasting 4–72 hours which has a minimum of two of the following four features:

1 Unilateral

2 Pulsating quality (varies with the heartbeat)

3 Moderate or severe intensity of pain

4 Aggravated by exercise.

In addition, the patient must experience nausea/vomiting and/or photophobia/phonophobia during the attack.

Auras typically occur 5–50 minutes before the headache and are visual, consisting of transient hemianopic disturbance or a spreading scotoma. There may also be focal neurological symptoms. Patients with prolonged auras should be referred for further investigation.

Headaches may change in nature over time, for example migraine may become chronic daily headache; in this case, treatment will need to be changed as appropriate.

Treatment algorithm

Start with simple oral analgesia, eg soluble ibuprofen (400–600 mg), aspirin (600–900 mg) or paracetamol. Patients should be advised to take analgesia as soon as possible after symptoms start, before gastric stasis develops.

If the patient complains of nausea, a prokinetic anti-emetic such as prochlorperazine (3 mg buccal tablet), domperidone (20 mg) or metoclopramide (10 mg) can be added; these help by increasing gastric emptying.

Rectal administration of diclofenac (100 mg) and domperidone (30 mg) may be more effective than oral medication; this should be tried as a second-line therapy.

If these measures fail, consider a triptan. Patients respond differently to the various triptans on offer, and if there is no response with the first one tried, it is worth changing formulation (eg to a nasal spray) or trying another triptan. Patients should be advised to take the triptan as soon as possible after the headache symptoms start but not until then, ie not during the aura. For all triptans except zolmitriptan, another dose should not be taken for the same migraine. If the migraine recurs however, then another dose can be taken, after an interval of at least 2 hours.

If an oral triptan is prescribed, a concomitant anti-emetic should be considered. Oral sumatriptan at a dose of 50 mg is often used as a first choice. The nasal spray offers no real advantage over oral medication if vomiting is a problem, as absorption will still be reduced. Sumatriptan also comes as a subcutaneous injection; this is particularly useful if a rapid effect is required.

Other appropriate choices include zolmitriptan 2.5 mg, either as a tablet or as Zomig Rapimelt®, an orodispersible tablet that is placed on the tongue and allowed to disperse, then swallowed. Zolmitriptan is licensed for adolescents.

Rizatriptan, 10-mg tablets or wafers, is useful if stronger treatment is required. Rizatriptan interacts with propranolol and in this case the dose should be reduced to 5 mg.

Almotriptan and eletriptan are still being evaluated in terms of their exact role in migraine management. Frovatriptan is the longest acting triptan on the market. Naratriptan has a relatively low efficacy and is most useful for patients who have significant adverse reactions to other triptans and in patients with frequent relapses.

Some patients find it beneficial to be given more than one type of triptan; for example, sumatriptan tablets and a zolmitriptan nasal spray. That way, if the tablet does not work for a particular migraine, the nasal spray can be tried.

Migraine prophylaxis

If the patient is getting frequent migraines that have an adverse effect on their lifestyle (eg more than four per month), it is then reasonable to consider prescribing a regular prophylactic medication for a period of about 4–6 months. The prophylactic medication can then be slowly tapered off over 2–3 weeks.

Beta-blockers such as propranolol or atenolol are usually the first choice unless there is a specific contraindication. The patient commonly starts with a very low dose of beta-blocker, eg 10 mg bd of propranolol, and then gradually has it titrated upwards until it has the desired effect. If one beta-blocker does not work, it is worth trying another. The patient should take the drug at an optimum dose for 1 month before treatment failure can be established. It is probably preferable to choose a relatively cardioselective beta-blocker initially, to minimise side-effects (eg atenolol 25 mg bd).

Amitriptyline 10–150 mg nocte is particularly useful when the migraine co-exists with tension-type headaches, chronic pain conditions or insomnia. Again, it should be started at a low dose and then titrated upwards. Amitriptyline does not have a licence for migraine prophylaxis.

Valproate 300–1000 mg bd is sometimes used as a second-line prophylactic treatment, but is contraindicated in pregnancy or when pregnancy is a possibility. Again, it is not licensed for migraine prophylaxis.

Pizotifen is also sometimes used, usually starting at a dose of 0.5 mg taken at night (it has a sedative action). Weight gain and increased appetite are common side-effects. It can be increased in increments of 0.5 mg every week until the patient is on 1.5 mg. Evidence for its efficacy is lacking, however, and it should not be used as a first-line treatment.

Verapamil is particularly good as prophylaxis for cluster headaches.

Feverfew is an option for patients who want to try a herbal alternative; it can be used at doses of 50–143 mg per day in adults. The primary care migraine guidelines (available at www.eguidelines.co.uk) state that herbal remedies should not be used alone, but only to complement conventional treatment.

If these measures do not work, there are other possibilities such as methysergide, which is highly effective but is associated with serious side-effects, including retroperitoneal fibrosis; for this reason, it should be initiated by a specialist.

Menstrual migraine

This is defined as attacks of migraine (without aura) that occur regularly around the onset of menstruation and at no other time. It is worth suggesting a trial of an NSAID at regular intervals for the duration of the menstrual period (eg mefenamic acid 500 mg tds–qds). Other options are estradiol gel (1.5 mg in 2.5 g) applied daily from day 3 for 7 days (no added progestogens are needed if the woman has regular cycles), the COCP or cerazette® (to inhibit ovulation). These measures should be tried for at least three cycles.

TENSION HEADACHES

These classically get worse during the course of the day and the headache is described as pressure or tightness, like a band around the head. It often affects the neck as well and is more common in sedentary people. Regular exercise and simple analgesia are often sufficient. However, if a patient complains of chronic tension headache (defined as having a headache on >15 days/month), they may need counselling about stress avoidance, or physiotherapy if there is musculoskeletal involvement.

MEDICATION-OVERUSE HEADACHE

Regular usage of simple analgesics (eg paracetamol ± codeine), triptans and possibly NSAIDs can result in medication-overuse headache. This usually only occurs in patients who regularly take three or more analgesic tablets daily or narcotics on more than 2 days a week. A diary of analgesic use can be very helpful. The headache is often worse first thing in the morning and is exacerbated by exercise. Symptoms resolve after the analgesics are withdrawn.

CLUSTER HEADACHES

These are rare, affecting 1/1000 men and 1/6000 women, and are more common in smokers. The most common type of cluster headache is the episodic type, in which extremely intense, strictly unilateral pain develops around one eye, often at night; attacks can come on daily or even several times a day, and last for 30 minutes to 2 hours. There is often associated lacrimation of the affected eye, which may be reddened; and nasal symptoms, such as blocked nose. Ptosis may also be present. These episodes can occur at regular intervals for a period of 6–12 weeks at a time, typically once every year or 2 years, often at the same time of year for many years or even decades.

There is a chronic form of cluster headache, in which there is no remission of pain between the clusters of headache, and a continuous milder background headache can develop that is present in-between attacks. Verapamil is often used as prophylaxis for patients with cluster headache and triptans may be helpful during an acute attack. These patients should usually be referred to a neurologist.

EPILEPSY

Patients with suspected epilepsy should be referred to a specialist as soon as possible, ideally within 2 weeks (NICE 2004). Treatment with anti-epileptic medication is generally recommended only after a second seizure. However, it may be instigated by a specialist after the first seizure if the patient has a neurological deficit, the EEG shows definite epileptic activity, brain imaging is abnormal, or if the patient is unable to accept the possibility that they may experience a second seizure.

For patients who have been diagnosed with epilepsy, an excellent source of information is the Joint Epilepsy Council of the UK and Ireland (www.jointepilepsycouncil.org.uk).

ANTI-EPILEPTIC MEDICATION

In general, monotherapy is preferred, and if the first-choice drug is ineffective, monotherapy with a different medication should be considered (NICE, 2004).

The usual first-line agents are carbamazepine and valproate; phenytoin is no longer routinely recommended. Newer anti-epileptic drugs include gabapentin, lamotrigine, levetiracetam, oxcarbazepine, tiagabine, topiramate and vigabatrin. They are only indicated if the patient has not been helped by conventional treatment with one of the older drugs, if the older drugs are contraindicated or if the patient is intolerant of them. Women of childbearing potential can also be offered one of the newer agents.

MONITORING ANTI-EPILEPTIC MEDICATION

Blood levels are only necessary in the following circumstances:

- To determine compliance with treatment
- If there is suspected toxicity
- If the dose of phenytoin needs to be adjusted
- If there is concern about interaction with other medications
- New-onset liver or kidney failure.

NICE recommends that all patients on enzyme-inducing drugs (carbamazepine, topiramate, oxcarbazepine, phenytoin and phenobarbital) should have routine bloods done every 2–5 years, including full blood count (FBC), urea and electrolytes (U&Es), liver function tests (LFTs), vitamin D levels and calcium.

STOPPING MEDICATION

The longer a patient has been seizure-free on treatment, the better their prognosis. The following factors increase the risk of relapse on withdrawal of medication:

- Age of onset of epilepsy >16 years

- Being on more than one anti-epileptic medication

- History of seizures while taking medication

- History of tonic-clonic or myoclonic seizures

- Abnormal EEG.

After 5 years of being seizure-free, a patient with one or two of the above risk factors has approximately a 20–30% risk of recurrent seizures on withdrawal of the medication (compared to a 10–15% risk if they continue taking it). After 10 years of being seizure-free, this risk drops to about 10% (or 5% if they continue taking the medication). The risk of a recurrent seizure is highest 9 months after withdrawal of treatment.

Anti-epileptic medication needs to be tapered off gradually over 2–3 months, usually under the supervision of a specialist. Only one medication should be stopped at a time.

CONTRACEPTIVE CHOICES FOR WOMEN ON ANTI-EPILEPTIC MEDICATION

For women taking hepatic enzyme-inducing anti-epileptic drugs (see above), the following considerations apply:

- The progesterone-only pill is not recommended.

- The progesterone implant is not recommended either.

- If the combined oral contraceptive pill is used, at a minimum initial dose of 50 micrograms. oestrogen is recommended. 'Tricycling' might be necessary if the woman experiences breakthrough bleeding.

- If the depot progesterone method is preferred, injections need to be given at intervals of 10 weeks instead of 12 weeks.

Women on anti-epileptic drugs should be advised that the doses of levonorgestrel used for emergency contraception need to be increased to 1.5 mg and 750 micrograms taken 12 hours apart.

EPILEPSY AND THE GMS CONTRACT

In order to be awarded maximum quality points, practices must achieve the following standards:

- There must be a register of all patients who are receiving anti-epileptic medication.

- 90% of patients aged 16 or over on drug treatment for epilepsy should have had a record of seizure frequency done in the past 15 months.

- 90% of patients aged 16 or over on treatment for epilepsy must have had a medication review done in the past 15 months.

- 70% of patients aged 16 or over on anti-epileptic medication should have been seizure-free for at least 12 months; this should have been recorded within the past 15 months.

PARKINSON'S DISEASE

Parkinson's syndrome (or parkinsonism) refers to the symptoms of tremor, rigidity (often 'cogwheel'), bradykinesia and difficulty in stopping or starting walking. Parkinson's disease (PD) is the most common cause of parkinsonism, but iatrogenic parkinsonism (due to treatment with dopamine antagonists) accounts for about 30% of cases. Cerebrovascular disease can also cause parkinsonism, usually of sudden onset. Early signs are loss of facial expression, general 'slowing down' of movements and unilateral loss of arm swing. Fatiguing occurs with repetitive movements such as opening and closing the hand, pronating and supinating the wrist or tapping the heel on the ground; this can be a useful diagnostic tool.

Treatment should be considered when the patient's symptoms begin to impact on their quality of life or if there is functional impairment. The most usual initial options are levodopa, monoamine oxidase type-B inhibitors such as selegiline, or dopamine agonists. Levodopa relieves symptoms in most patients, but long-term use is associated with motor complications such as involuntary movements (dyskinesia), as well as a shortened response to each dose (wearing-off phenomenon) and unpredictable 'on-off' fluctuations. Using a dopamine agonist or selegiline initially may reduce the need for levodopa; indeed, a recent systematic review (*British Medical Journal* 2004; **329**: 593) concluded that selegiline reduces disability, the need for levodopa and the incidence of motor fluctuations. Because of these different options, treatment should usually be initiated by a specialist or by a GP with a special interest in PD. In general, dopamine agonists are used as first-line treatment in the younger patient who does not have other serious co-morbidities.

Approximately 25% of patients with PD will develop dementia, and up to 50% may become depressed. Antidepressant medication can interact with PD drugs or worsen parkinsonian symptoms and should only be initiated with guidance from a specialist. Selective serotonin reuptake inhibitors (SSRIs) and mirtazapine may be the best choices.

Essential tremor	Parkinson's disease
Worse on movement	Rest tremor, 'pill-rolling'
Relieved by alcohol and by propranolol (eg 10–40 mg bd)	Not affected by alcohol or beta-blockers
Often bilateral	Usually unilateral onset
Younger patient, often with family history of tremor	Older patient (average age 65)

Table 9.1: Differentiating essential tremor from Parkinson's disease tremor

CHAPTER 10
OBSTETRICS

CHAPTER 10
OBSTETRICS

ANTENATAL AND POSTNATAL CARE

SCHEDULE OF VISITS (NICE 2003)

Gestation	Purpose of visit
8–12 weeks	Booking visit. Patient should be referred to hospital, given information on Down's syndrome screening, smoking cessation and dietary advice, including alcohol reduction. She should receive information about the schedule of antenatal visits and ultrasound scans. Booking bloods (including FBC, blood grouping, screening tests for HIV, hepatitis, syphilis and rubella immunity) and a urine culture should be sent off. If nuchal scanning is not offered, the woman should be given an appointment for a dating scan
12–16 weeks	Down's syndrome screening
16 weeks	Information on accessing parent education, antenatal and breastfeeding workshops. Review of blood test results
20 weeks	Anomaly scan
25 weeks*	Routine care (fetal growth, blood pressure, urine dipstick and benefit forms, eg Mat B1, FW8, Sure Start)
28 weeks	Routine care. Routine bloods to screen for anaemia and atypical red cell alloantibodies. Discuss infant feeding, health promotion and smoking cessation. Confirm access to parent education

31 weeks*	Routine care and review, discuss blood results
34 weeks	Routine care
36 weeks	Routine care, including checking presentation of the baby (this should not be attempted before 36 weeks as examination may be inaccurate and cause anxiety). Offer external cephalic version if indicated. Any suspected malpresentation should be confirmed with ultrasound
38 weeks	Routine care and information leaflet regarding 41-week visit
40 weeks*	Routine care
41 weeks	Routine care, discuss labour plans and possibility of induction

*Visits for primips only

Table 10.1: Schedule of antenatal visits

NICE recommends only ten antenatal visits for women in their first (uncomplicated) pregnancy and seven in subsequent pregnancies, as there is no evidence that care is improved by the woman being seen more frequently. Routine glucose tolerance testing is no longer recommended unless the woman is at high risk (eg South Asian, family history of type 2 diabetes, polycystic ovarian disease (PCOS) or obese). Women do not need to be seen by a consultant if the pregnancy is uncomplicated. An early scan is recommended (ideally between 10 and 13 weeks, possibly combined with the nuchal scan), to confirm dates and exclude multiple pregnancies.

DOWN'S SYNDROME TESTING

It is currently recommended that all obstetric units should be able to provide either nuchal translucency measurement (done between 11 and 14 weeks) or biochemical screening (done between 14 and 20 weeks) for their clients, regardless of age. However, by 2007, the aim is to offer women more accurate testing, either with the combined test (using nuchal translucency and biochemistry at 11–14 weeks) or with the quadruple biochemistry test at 14–20 weeks. Eventually, a combination of first and second trimester screening will be employed, whereby the detection rate may be as high as 95%; this is known as the 'integrated test' and consists of the nuchal scan and a blood test for pregnancy-associated plasma protein A (PAPP-A) and human chorionic gonadotrophin (hCG) between 11 and 14 weeks and a blood test for alpha-fetoprotein (AFP), estriol (uE3) and inhibin A at 14–20 weeks.

DIETARY ADVICE

Women should take 400 µg folic acid during the first 12 weeks of pregnancy (or 5 mg per day if they are on anti-epileptic medication, if they have already had a child with spina bifida or if they have diabetes mellitus, coeliac disease or other malabsorption syndromes). Other vitamin supplements are rarely needed, although a small percentage of women with inadequate diets or lack of exposure to sunlight may need additional vitamin D; this can be obtained free of charge if they receive Income Support or income-based Jobseeker's Allowance.

Anaemia in pregnancy is defined as a haemoglobin level of <11 g/dl initially or <10.5 g/dl at 28 weeks. These women may need iron supplements.

Alcohol should be limited to no more than 7 units per week, spread out over the week.

Most women gain between 10kg and 12.5 kg during pregnancy. As always, a sensible balanced diet, rich in fruit and vegetables, is recommended. However, the following specific dietary advice should be given:

- Dairy products are a good source of calcium (ideally the low-fat varieties), as are oily fish with edible bones (eg sardines), bread, green vegetables and nuts. Pregnant women on Income Support or income-based Jobseeker's Allowance can get seven pints of cow's milk free per week. Unpasteurised milk and milk products are **not** recommended (eg some goat's milk and sheep's milk).

- All fruit and vegetables should be washed carefully, to reduce the risk of acquiring toxoplasmosis.

- All meat and poultry should be cooked thoroughly and careful hygiene maintained when preparing raw meat; again, this is to reduce the risk of getting toxoplasmosis.

- Eggs should be cooked properly to reduce the risk of catching *Salmonella*; soft-boiled eggs are not recommended.

- All pâtés and mould-ripened soft cheeses should be avoided, as should blue-veined cheeses such as stilton; this is because of potential *Listeria* infection. Exceptions are the soft cheeses made from pasteurised milk, such as cottage cheese, cheese spreads and mozzarella; these are fine in pregnancy.

- All ready-made meals should be heated through thoroughly.

- Liver should be avoided because of its high vitamin A content.

- Women who have a personal history of atopy (eg eczema, asthma or hayfever), or who have an affected partner should avoid peanuts and foods containing peanuts.

- Shark, marlin and swordfish contain high levels of mercury, which may affect the fetus.

ANTENATAL INFECTIONS

Toxoplasmosis

Toxoplasmosis is caused by the *Toxoplasma gondii* parasite, which can be acquired by eating undercooked meat and by coming into contact with cat faeces. Pregnant women should be advised not to change cat-litter trays or to handle soil that might have been contaminated. All fruit and vegetables should be washed thoroughly and rubber gloves should be used when gardening. There is currently insufficient evidence to propose nationwide screening; there is no clear proof that antenatal treatment of women with presumed toxoplasmosis reduces congenital transmission (*Cochrane Review*, Issue 4, 2004).

Women who have 'flu-like' symptoms in pregnancy or who believe themselves to be at significant risk from toxoplasmosis can be offered serological testing. A negative result implies that the patient has never had toxoplasmosis and is not immune. One in three women has a positive result, usually because of previous exposure; in this case, the blood sample is sent to a reference laboratory to exclude current infection. It is thought that it takes between 4 and 6 weeks for toxoplasmosis to pass from mother to baby and the risk of congenital infection depends on when the woman was affected. If infection occurred shortly before conception (ie 2–3 months before), there is a very low risk of transmission (<1%). Most affected fetuses will miscarry at this stage. If infection occurs in the first trimester, the transmission rate is about 15%. This rate increases as the pregnancy progresses and is as high as 65% by the third trimester. Most affected babies will be symptomatic. The severest disabilities are found in children whose mothers were infected early on in pregnancy, and include hydrocephalus and retinochoroiditis. Children whose mothers were infected in the third trimester often appear healthy at birth, but most will develop symptoms later on (months or even years afterwards), usually visual problems. Amniocentesis testing can be offered to affected women. Treatment with spiramycin reduces the risk of transmission from mother to baby, but cannot prevent damage to a fetus who is already infected.

Chickenpox

Approximately 90% of adults in the UK are immune to varicella zoster and are IgG-positive (*Ir J Med Sci* 2000; 169: 288); this figure is lower in women from tropical and subtropical regions. The incubation period of varicella ranges from 10 days to 21 days. Patients are contagious from 48 hours before the appearance of the rash until the vesicles crust over.

Overall, approximately 0.3% of pregnancies in the UK are complicated by chickenpox infection. Infection may be more severe in pregnancy and 10% of affected women go on to develop pneumonia. Babies born to women who become infected with varicella before 20 weeks' gestation have a 1–2% risk of developing the fetal varicella syndrome (FVS). This is a disastrous outcome, characterised by neurological disability (microcephaly, cortical atrophy and severe developmental delay), visual defects (including retinochoroiditis, congenital cataracts and microphthalmia), skin scarring and limb hypoplasia.

Maternal chickenpox infection between 20 and 36 weeks' gestation does not appear to result in an adverse outcome for the fetus, except that the child may be at increased risk of developing shingles in the first few years of life.

Between 36 weeks' gestation and term, maternal infection may result in the baby becoming infected with chickenpox (officially called 'varicella infection of the newborn'), but is not associated with FVS. The closer the infection occurs to the time of delivery, the greater the risk of severe infection in the newborn, with a significant mortality rate, especially if the baby is born within 7 days of the onset of the mother's rash. In this case, there are also serious maternal risks, including thrombocytopenia and disseminated intravascular coagulation (DIC). Hospital admission is necessary and intravenous aciclovir is usually administered.

The following measures can be considered to prevent FVS and varicella infection of the newborn (*RCOG Guideline* No 13, July 2001):

- In the USA and certain European countries, women planning to become pregnant who are known to be non-immune are offered the varicella vaccine. However, it is not licensed for this indication in the UK.

- Women booking in for antenatal care should be advised to avoid contact with chickenpox if there is no clear history of previous exposure.

- Pregnant women who are unsure of their immune status and who come into contact with chickenpox should be offered serological testing for varicella zoster IgG; most labs will be able to provide a result within 24 hours if they know it is an urgent request. If the IgG is negative, varicella zoster immunoglobulin (VZIG) should be given as soon as possible, and certainly within 10 days of the contact. If an IgG taken within 10 days of the contact is positive, the patient must have had pre-existing immunity.

- Pregnant women who actually develop chickenpox should be given aciclovir within 24 hours of the onset of the rash if they are at more than 20 weeks of gestation; there is no evidence that it is effective if the rash has been present for more than 24 hours. VZIG is not effective in patients with established chickenpox. Pneumonia is a potential complication, and women should be asked to report any new respiratory symptoms to their doctor as soon as possible. Women who develop chickenpox in the first 20 weeks will need referral for detailed ultrasound examination and possibly amniotic fluid testing.

- Maternal shingles does not pose a risk to the fetus or neonate. Non-immune pregnant women should avoid coming into close contact with somebody who has shingles, although the risk of catching chickenpox in this situation is low unless infection is extensive or the patient with shingles is immunocompromised.

Parvovirus B19

Parvovirus B19 is the cause of fifth disease (also known as 'slapped cheek' disease and erythema infectiosum). It is very common in the UK and 50–60% of adults have evidence of past infection. It can present as a minor febrile illness with or without a rash; if present, this often starts on the cheeks, then spreads to the trunk. Clinically, it is difficult to distinguish from rubella. More serious disease occasionally occurs, for example aplastic crises in patients with sickle cell disease.

Infection in the first 20 weeks of pregnancy can lead to miscarriage (9% additional risk) and to hydrops fetalis (3% risk if infection is acquired between weeks 9 and 20, of which about half will die). These effects on the fetus usually occur about 3–5 weeks after the onset of maternal infection. Permanent congenital abnormality is not commonly associated with intrauterine parvovirus B19 infection, but persistent neonatal infection and anaemia do occasionally occur.

Any pregnant woman who has a non-vesicular rash herself or who has been in significant contact (ie either face-to-face contact or in the same room for >15 minutes) with somebody with a rash should be tested for parvovirus B19 and rubella infection, unless there is already documented evidence of immunity; serological testing is easy to organise. Women who test negative for parvovirus IgG and IgM should have a repeat test 1 month after the time of contact. Those with proved parvovirus B19 infection in the first 20 weeks of pregnancy should be followed up by serial ultrasound and referred to a regional specialist centre for consideration of fetal blood sampling and intrauterine transfusion if hydrops fetalis is detected. (*Communicable Disease and Public Health* Vol 5, No 1, March 2002)

Genital herpes

Neonatal herpes infection is rare in the UK (incidence 1.65/100 000 live births per year (*J Antimicrobial Chemother* 2000; 45 Suppt 3: 7–13) but potentially very serious. The risk is highest if the mother acquires the infection for the first time during the later stages of her pregnancy. Oral aciclovir is often used for women who develop a first episode of genital herpes during pregnancy (*RCOG Clinical Guideline* No 30, March 2002).

Caesarean section is recommended for all women presenting with their first episode of genital herpes at the time of delivery (or within 6 weeks of the expected date of delivery), but not for women presenting in the first or second trimester. For women presenting with recurrent genital herpes at the time of delivery, the risk to the baby is small and elective Caesarean section is not mandatory. Operative delivery is not recommended if there is a recurrent episode of genital herpes occurring at any other time during pregnancy.

Group B *Streptococcus*

Group B *Streptococcus* (GBS) is the most common cause of severe infection in neonates within the first 7 days of life. In other countries such as the USA, routine screening of pregnant women with a vaginal or rectal swab at 35–37 weeks of gestation is recommended and affected women are given intrapartum iv penicillin or ampicillin.

Approximately 25% of women of childbearing age in the UK are GBS carriers (*J Antimicrobial Chemother*; 1986; 18: 59–65), so if routine screening and treatment were introduced, more than 200 000 women per year would receive intravenous antibiotics during labour. In more than 99.9% of cases this would be unnecessary, with the potential for adverse drug reactions occurring as a result; it has been estimated that at least 7000 women would need to be treated to prevent one neonatal death.

In general practice, women are sometimes incidentally found to be GBS carriers. In these cases, oral antibiotics at the time of diagnosis are **not** recommended; giving them does not reduce the likelihood of the woman becoming recolonised at the time of delivery (*Am J Obstet Gynaecol* 1979;

135: 1062–5). The decision of whether or not to give intrapartum antibiotics is more difficult. If the swab was taken at 35–37 weeks, there is a 0.2% chance of the baby being affected, although this risk may be greater if the swab was taken from the upper vagina or if there is GBS present in the urine. In any case, the final decision will be made by an obstetrician, and the main responsibility of the GP is to record the swab result in the woman's antenatal records and to explain the situation to her.

PERINEAL TEARS (RCOG GUIDELINE NO 29 JULY 2001)

All women who have had a third- or fourth-degree tear should be followed up for 12 months after delivery, as symptoms may not appear straight away. If the woman is suffering from faecal incontinence, she should be offered an endoanal ultrasound and anorectal manometry. Secondary sphincter repair can be considered. Subsequent deliveries may worsen symptoms of faecal incontinence, or cause them to develop, so elective Caesarean section may be an option.

Broad-spectrum antibiotics and laxatives (usually an osmotic laxative such as lactulose, in combination with a bulking agent such as Fybogel®) are often prescribed after a third- or fourth-degree tear has been repaired: this is to reduce the incidence of wound dehiscence and postoperative infection. Metronidazole is usually included as part of the treatment, in order to cover anaerobic infection from faecal matter.

POSTNATAL EXERCISES

Pelvic floor exercises are very important (see Chapter 7, Gynaecology).

The following exercises to strengthen the abdominal muscles can be started as soon after the birth as the mother wishes:

1 She should lie on her back with her head on a pillow, arms by her side and knees bent. She should press the small of her back into the bed whilst drawing in her abdominal muscles; this flattened position should be held for 4 seconds and repeated as often as possible.

2 The next stage is to do step 1 without a pillow.

3 After this, she should lift her head and reach towards her knees with outstretched hands, whilst lying in the flattened position. A twisting exercise, whereby she reaches with one hand to the opposite ankle whilst lying in the same position can also be attempted.

If at any time there is evidence of a divarication of the abdominal muscles, these exercises should be stopped and the woman referred to a physiotherapist.

CHAPTER 11
OPHTHALMOLOGY

CHAPTER 11
OPHTHALMOLOGY

BLEPHARITIS

Many patients suffer from troublesome, recurrent attacks of blepharitis. A good preventative strategy is to clean the eyes regularly once or twice a day with diluted baby shampoo (one part shampoo to four parts water), using a cotton bud. An alternative to baby shampoo is a teaspoon of baking soda diluted in a pint of water. Exacerbations may be caused by superimposed *Staphylococcus* infection, in which case a 1-week course of chloramphenicol ointment (bd) may be necessary; this should also be applied with a cotton bud. Occasionally, patients with severe posterior blepharitis occurring in association with acne may need 3–6 months of oral doxycycline.

EXCESS LACRIMATION

Causes include:

- Overproduction of tears, eg due to corneal irritation from an ectropion (out-turning of the eyelid) or entropion (in-turning of the eyelid). These conditions usually need surgical correction, but topical lubricants can provide temporary relief. Patients with entropion, whose in-turning eyelashes are causing abrasion of the cornea, may be helped by taping the eyelid into mild ectropion. Ectropions and entropions usually affect the lower eyelids.

- Overproduction of tears for another reason, eg hayfever, blepharitis, corneal foreign body.

- Impaired drainage from a partially blocked nasolacrimal duct. Approximately 20% of neonates have imperforate or stenosed ducts and produce ocular discharge which simply consists of mucus and is not infected. Parents should be reassured that most children are better by the time they reach the age of 1 year. They should be advised to massage their baby's lacrimal sac four times a day. Topical antibiotics are only indicated if there is evidence of infective conjunctivitis.

The nasolacrimal duct can also become stenosed with age (age-related lacrimal drainage obstruction). These patients may have intermittent swelling of their lacrimal sacs (lacrimal sac mucocoele) and are more likely to develop dacryocystitis (see below).

Surgery is possible for patients with troublesome symptoms.

DACRYOCYSTITIS (LACRIMAL SAC INFECTION)

The patient will present with inflammation medially, over the lacrimal sac. There may be a previous history of excess watering of the affected eye, due to a partially blocked nasolacrimal duct. Systemic and topical antibiotics are necessary and the patient will need to be referred if their symptoms do not settle quickly because there is a danger that a lacrimal sac abscess may form.

CHALAZION

A chalazion is a granuloma of a lipid-secreting meibomian gland in the eyelid and it will usually resolve spontaneously. The patient should be advised to use hot compresses (a flannel soaked in warm water) and topical antibiotic ointment may be prescribed if there is evidence of superimposed infection. Chalazia persisting for more than 6 months can be referred for excision if the patient so wishes.

Recurrent chalazia may occur in association with blepharitis and acne rosacea.

STYE

A stye is an infection of a lash follicle and may be easily confused with an infected chalazion. It can be treated with hot compresses and topical antibiotic ointment.

PTERYGIUM

A Pterigium is a triangular-shaped lesion that begins outside the limbus and may cross over it onto the cornea. It is almost always found on the nasal aspect of the eye and is commonly bilateral. They are probably caused by excess UV light. Common presenting symptoms include redness, soreness and dryness (exacerbated by sunlight, wind, air-conditioning and smoke), although some patients are predominantly concerned about the appearance of their eye. Visual disturbance is uncommon but can occur with severe disease. These patients should usually see an optician initially for correction of refraction, but a minority may need referral for excision.

Most pterygia can be managed in primary care; patients should be given lifestyle advice on avoidance of sunlight, smoke, etc, and can be prescribed topical lubricants such as hypromellose.

Differential diagnoses include pingueculae, which are small bilateral grey, white or yellowish nodules that occur at the 3 o'clock and 9 o'clock positions of the eye, just outside the limbus and which are usually found in elderly patients. They are treated conservatively. Squamous cell carcinoma of the conjunctiva is very rare and presents as a unilateral irregular, rounded lesion, with a rough uneven surface.

BACTERIAL CONJUNCTIVITIS

Bacterial conjunctivitis is usually bilateral and the patient may complain of sticky eyes (especially in the morning) which are red and gritty. Associated eyelid oedema is common. Sufferers should be prescribed topical antibiotics if the infection is severe (usually chloramphenicol) and be advised to clean their eyelids and eyes with cooled boiled water twice a day. The bottle containing the topical antibiotics should not touch the eye when it is being applied. Artificial tears can help to soothe the eye.

Without treatment, symptoms may be marked for about a week, then resolve over the course of 2–3 weeks. Conjunctivitis is highly contagious and patients should not share towels, facecloths or pillowcases and should wash their hands every time they touch their eyes.

Allergy to topical antibiotics can develop: this usually presents with itching and eyelid oedema and is the most common cause for apparent 'non-resolution'. The patient often shows an initial improvement when the antibiotic is first prescribed, before deteriorating again. Symptoms commonly resolve within 24 hours of stopping treatment.

Conjunctivitis occurring in contact lens wearers can be potentially sight-threatening. Patients with mild infection with no visual loss are usually treated in primary care, but need to be followed up carefully and referred if it does not improve within a few days. The patient should not use lenses for at least 1 week after the infection has fully resolved and will need a fresh pair when they do resume wear.

Contact lens wearers (particularly those who don't clean their lenses often enough) may develop a protozoal infection called *Acanthamoeba* keratitis. This usually presents with ocular pain or 'aching'. Swabs are negative and symptoms are more pronounced than signs. Such patients should be referred to an ophthalmologist.

ALLERGIC CONJUNCTIVITIS

This is often seasonal and responds to oral or topical antihistamines (such as azelastine). Topical mast cell stabilisers such as sodium cromoglicate are also used, but may take up to 2 weeks to work.

MACULAR DEGENERATION

Age-related macular degeneration (AMD) is the leading cause of blindness in the UK. Central vision is affected, with peripheral vision remaining intact. Chronic, slowly-progressing disease is called dry AMD. Wet AMD implies choroidal neovascularisation and necessitates an urgent referral; treatment with pholodynamic therapy is possible for wet disease but not for dry disease. Patients with known dry AMD should be asked to test their eyes regularly (eg on alternate days) by covering up each eye in turn and looking at a straight object such as a door frame or crossword. If straight lines look curved, they should see a doctor as soon as possible; this may indicate the onset of wet AMD. In this case, urgent referral is important, because ideally treatment with photodynamic therapy should take place within 2 weeks of the onset of symptoms.

There is limited evidence that high-dose vitamins A, C, E and zinc and copper supplements help to prevent wet disease from occurring; these are found in multivitamin preparations such as ICAPS® or OCUVITE®, but cannot be prescribed under the NHS.

BLINDNESS

Patients who wish to be registered as blind need to have form BD8 filled in; this is usually done by an ophthalmologist. Most people who have vision of <3/60 Snellen qualify. People who have vision of between 3/60 and 6/60 with a very contracted field of vision are also eligible, as are those with vision >6/60 with a very contracted field of vision, especially if the contraction is in the lower part of the field. Patients with homonymous hemianopia or bitemporal hemianopia should **not** be certified as blind if their central vision is ≥6/18 Snellen, but they can usually be registered as being partially sighted.

Many of these patients will benefit from being referred to the Low Vision Clinic at their local hospital; they may be offered free low vision aids through the Hospital Eye Service. Social Services involvement is also important, in terms of helping the patient to remain at home and to arrange mobility training. Partially sighted patients are eligible for Social Services assistance as well, but may not qualify for the same financial benefits. People can apply to the Guide Dogs for the Blind Association for their own guide dog.

There are various charitable institutions which can also offer help, including Action for Blind People, the Royal National Institute for the Blind and the Partially Sighted Society (if the patient still has some residual vision); see Useful Contact Information, p. 329 for details.

CHAPTER 12
ORTHOPAEDICS

CHAPTER 12
ORTHOPAEDICS

FRACTURE CARE

Most patients with fractures will present to the Emergency Department and be followed up in a fracture clinic. However, if a patient presents in primary care, it is worth knowing that fracture clinics are usually held every day and referral to the clinic is easy to make. Usually the on-call registrar will be happy to answer any simple questions, or make a fracture clinic appointment for a few days' time, but they are often 'in theatre' (!), so here is a basic guide to fracture management.

BASIC AIM

The bone will usually heal eventually. The trick is to make sure it heals in an 'acceptable' position. For a tibia, this may be with only 50% of the bone surfaces touching, whereas for a fracture through a joint, the position has to be within a millimetre of normal. Even if the fracture is in an acceptable position to begin with, that position can be lost before the bone has healed. This is usually the result of weight-bearing or lifting with the limb, or of the action of muscles that attach to the bone. Visits to the Fracture Clinic are made to check the position in the earlier stages of healing, and, later on, to assess whether there is sufficient healing to allow removal of any external splint to the bone, such as a plaster cast.

TIMINGS – HOW LONG A BONE TAKES TO HEAL

There is a very simple rule of thumb: the quickest bone to heal is a child's arm (about 3 weeks) and that time is doubled for an adult and doubled again if the fracture is below the waist. An adult tibial fracture is therefore 'healed' after about 12 weeks. Of course, many factors slow this process down or potentially stop it from happening altogether, especially smoking and the usual delaying factors to wound healing, such as infection or poor blood supply.

It is worth bearing in mind that these timings are quite arbitrary. For example, it is actually very hard to manipulate an old lady's Colles' fracture after only 3 weeks. However, her cast will still be kept on for 6 weeks altogether, as the fracture remains mobile enough to 'creep' and lose the desired position. For the same reason, a boisterous child is often kept in plaster for 1–2 weeks longer than the theoretical 'healing time' for their fracture.

As yet, no process has been found to reliably speed up fracture healing, although claims have been made for ultrasound and pulsed electromagnetic fields. These are not in routine use in the UK.

WHAT TO TELL THE PATIENT WITH A FRACTURE OR DISLOCATION

The plaster is designed to leave certain joints free; these joints should be moved as much as possible.

Patients who have dislocated a joint need to be careful with specific movements for at least 2 weeks, until the soft tissues have healed sufficiently to prevent re-dislocation. Essentially, the movement that caused the dislocation in the first place should be avoided, eg patients with anterior dislocation of the shoulder should avoid external rotation.

Patients with fractures that are not treated in a plaster (eg fifth metatarsal fractures, radial head fractures) should be advised to do as much as is comfortable. Gentle movement will help to prevent the stiffness that occurs following plaster treatment. Pain should be their guide and as long as they stop when it begins to get sore and the pain resolves soon afterwards, there should be no adverse consequence in terms of healing. Tubigrip® should be removed at night. Putting Tubigrip® back on can be difficult, so ask the patient to roll it off and then roll it back on again in the morning, taking care to avoid creases. If a patient cannot tolerate Tubigrip®, then leaving it off will not significantly impair healing, although oedema may be more of a problem.

As for the usual question of 'When can I go back to ...?', there is no evidence-based answer. As a guide, after 3 weeks a child's arm may well be healed enough to have a plaster removed, but care should still be taken for a further month. Direct trauma and twisting are likely to cause a re-fracture, so contact sports and bicycle riding should be modified accordingly. The muscle wasting and joint stiffness that result from a period in a plaster cast will often make sports too painful anyway. Bone responds to use and so it is best to do as much as is comfortable when the plaster is removed and the very sporty child can be encouraged to maintain fitness with swimming, gym work, etc and avoid direct trauma until the muscle strength has been regained and bone remodelling has taken place.

SLINGS

A broad arm sling is designed to take the weight of an arm, thereby relieving the shoulder and enforcing a degree of elevation. It can therefore be removed for sleeping or exercising. It is the treatment of choice for a fractured clavicle.

A collar and cuff holds the wrist and leaves the elbow free. This gives an axial traction force to the upper arm, which is why it is used to maintain the alignment of humeral fractures. Because it is being used to keep the fracture aligned, the collar and cuff should be worn at all times (unless the patient is lying down) and the patient needs to be told not to adjust it 'to support the elbow' as this will obviously remove the traction force.

TYPES OF PLASTER

Plaster comes in two types. The old-fashioned plaster of Paris is used in the initial management of a fracture. The patient is given a backslab, to allow the soft tissues room to swell and then to allow the swelling to recede without the plaster becoming too tight or loose. After the initial week following the injury, most patients return to clinic to have the backslab changed to a fibreglass cast, which is lighter, stronger and more durable. They will also usually have an X-ray to check that the initial fracture position is still satisfactory. The exception is when the fracture has needed to be manipulated and held with a cast applied in theatre. In this case, only plaster of Paris can be moulded to produce a correctly shaped cast that holds the unstable fracture properly and this cast is not usually changed after a week.

PRACTICAL PROBLEMS WITH PLASTER

A plaster is inconvenient. Even the fibreglass ones are not waterproof; the layer of cotton wool on the skin becomes waterlogged and uneven, resulting in rolls and pressure areas. A plastic bag and tape is one solution, but there are also proprietary products available from every plaster room or fracture clinic that produce a watertight seal sufficient to allow bathing and even swimming. These cost between £10 and £20 depending on size. Under no circumstances should anything be put down inside a plaster to scratch the skin underneath. Strangely, scratching the outside often helps, as does avoiding excess heat or sweating. Pressure sores can develop under a cast, and have been known to lead to full-thickness tissue loss and amputation. **If there is an increase in the pain after the plaster has been put on, then it is unlikely to be due to the fracture, and may represent a pressure sore or infection (especially if there is a wound). Increased pain is therefore a reason to remove the cast.** Plaster rooms are open most days and plaster technicians are always available in working hours. They are also often needed to repair or reinforce a cast that has been on for a few weeks.

INTERNAL FIXATION

The metalwork needs to hold the fracture fragments in the correct position until the bone has healed. Once this has happened, the metal has done its job and could in theory be removed, although this is rarely done in practice. If there is a problem (eg metalwork around joints often works loose), removal is very easy. It is unlikely that having metal in situ will cause ongoing pain. Often, any pain experienced is due to secondary osteoarthritis or soft-tissue scarring from the injury. Patients should be aware that there is a 30% chance of nerve injury when metalwork is removed. There is an argument for removing metal from children (whose bones are still growing) and from very active patients, who are likely to re-fracture the bone in the future. Once metal has been removed, the remaining screw holes are a weak point until they fill in with new bone (in about 2–3 months), and so care needs to be taken in avoiding direct trauma and subsequent re-fracture. One important exception is the diastasis screw used in fixing some ankle fractures. This needs to be in place for 6 weeks to allow the soft tissues that hold the distal tibia and fibula together to heal. When the ankle bears weight, this area moves and the screw will break. Some surgeons accept this, but most will want to remove the diastasis screw 6 weeks after the fracture is fixed, so that the patient can begin to safely weight-bear.

Kirschner wires (usually called K-wires) are 1- to 2-mm-diameter wires that are drilled through the skin and bone to hold an unstable fracture fragment in place. They are left outside the skin and the patient (and practice nurse) should be warned about this before the dressings are removed. Like plaster of Paris, they are removed when the fracture has healed sufficiently that it no longer needs any external support. They are removed in clinic with no anaesthetic or sedation needed, using a pair of pliers.

External fixators and their larger brother, the Ilizarov circular frame, are also external scaffolds with pins through the skin into the fracture fragments. Again, they are left on until the fracture has achieved sufficient strength that it no longer needs supporting. From a GP's point of view, care needs to be taken to make sure the pin sites are not becoming infected. Daily dressing with Jelonet® or a dry dressing is often needed. **Infection needs prompt treatment with antibiotics**, as the wire is both a foreign body and a pathway for the bacteria to travel to the fracture site and cause osteomyelitis. The screws should be kept tight and most patients should have been given an 11-mm spanner for this purpose. For limb lengthening and other reconstructive procedures, the patient will have to turn one of the screws periodically. A nurse specialist will have taught them how to do all this, but if you are called upon, then tightening is clockwise! Frames are also removed in clinic with pliers, but a large frame on an anxious child will sometimes need a quick general anaesthetic.

Infection in a fracture fixation wound is a disaster. It will rapidly progress to osteomyelitis and the bone is unlikely to heal before the wound breaks down completely. Suspected infection should be treated early and aggressively. Wounds underneath plaster casts are a particular problem, so any increase in pain should be a reason to cut a window in the cast to inspect the wound. Emergency departments, operating theatres and plaster rooms in hospital will have the necessary equipment. Windows are also cut to allow access for suture removal.

PHYSIOTHERAPY

After any fracture, soft tissues will be inflamed and scarred and the patient may need a course of physiotherapy until full function has returned. Careful notice should be taken of any caveats from the treating surgeon regarding restrictions in weight-bearing status or active versus passive physiotherapy. The wait for physiotherapy is often a problem; the following exercises act as a guide as to what can be taught while the patient is waiting for the initial physiotherapy consultation, after their plaster has been removed. The exercises may also be useful for patients with other conditions, as explained below.

ANKLES

The exercises shown in Figure 12.1 will help after a sprain (once the acute phase is over) or after a fracture, by strengthening the musculature around the joint.

- Walk on tiptoe for 30 seconds.

- Walk on heels for 30 seconds.

- Rest leg on a footstool and hold calf to isolate ankle. Then draw large letters A, B, C, etc in the air with the big toe.

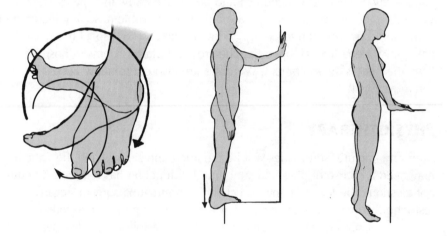

Figure 12.1 Ankle exercises

KNEE

The exercises in Figure 12.2 will help to build up weakened quadriceps, which has occurred secondary to a fracture or to osteoarthritis.

- Sit in a chair with a weight taped to the foot. Bend and straighten the knee.

- Sit in a chair and use the good leg to push the ankle and foot of the bad leg beneath the chair, to increase knee flexion.

- Sit in a chair with the foot resting on a footstool and use the hands to gently press the knee towards full extension.

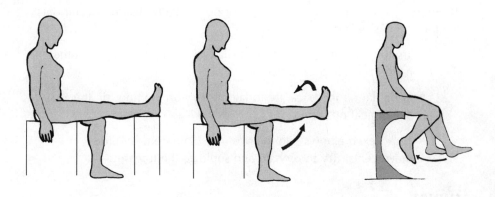

Figure 12.2 Knee exercises

SHOULDER

These exercises are primarily intended for post-fracture patients once clinical and radiographic union has been achieved.

- Sit in a chair and lean sideways with the arm straight and pointing towards the floor. Ask the patient to draw imaginary circles on the floor keeping their arm straight. Draw larger and larger circles.

- Hold a broomstick horizontally in both hands. Raise it above the head, thereby using the good arm to increase forward flexion of the bad shoulder.

ELBOW

These exercises are primarily intended for post-fracture patients, again once the fracture has united.

- Try to place the hand on the ipsilateral shoulder, using the other hand to gently push if necessary.

- Lying flat on the back, try to lay the arm on the floor (in the anatomical position).

- Tuck flexed elbows into the ribs (to isolate from shoulder movements). Try to pronate and supinate the forearm.

WRIST

These exercises are primarily intended for post-fracture patients.

- Hold the hands, palms together, above the head. Slowly bring the hands down, keeping the palms together (the namaste greeting)

- Hold the hands back to back by the groin or held out in front of the body. Slowly bring the hands towards the body, keeping the wristwatch areas touching and metacarpophalangeal joints (MCPJs) straight.

- Tuck flexed elbows into the ribs (to isolate from shoulder movements). Try to pronate and supinate the forearm.

TWISTED ANKLES

A surprising number of 'twisted' ankles turn out to be fractured on X-ray. The Ottawa System (Stiell I G, Greenberg G H, McKnight R D, Nair R C, McDowell I, Worthington J R, 'A study to develop clinical decision rules for the use of radiography in acute ankle injuries' *Ann Emerg Med* 1992; 21: 384–390) gives a guide as to who needs to be sent for an X-ray: patients with bony tenderness at the posterior edge or tip of the lateral or medial malleolus and patients who cannot weight-bear after the injury and who cannot walk four steps when assessed in the Emergency Department should have an ankle X-ray. Patients who have pain in their midfoot in conjunction with tenderness at the base of the fifth metatarsal or bone tenderness at the navicular, or who cannot weight-bear after the accident and when assessed in the Emergency Department should have a foot X-ray. Even this is not 100% sensitive. For a ligament sprain, simple RICE protocol (Rest, Ice, Compression, Elevation) advice will usually suffice. Crutches (and wheelchairs) can be rented from the Red Cross for a nominal fee if mobility is a problem. A severe ankle sprain may need enforced resting by being placed in a below-knee walking cast. The adage that a sprain is sometimes more painful than a fracture and can take longer to heal is true. Severe repeated sprains damage and stretch the supportive ankle ligaments and make further sprains more likely. Often a patient may need a long course of physiotherapy to develop the muscles around the ankle to a level at which they can support the ankle, and retraining is needed in balance and gait after recurrent sprains have destroyed the proprioception from the joint.

THE ACUTELY PAINFUL KNEE

ACUTE INJURIES

Twisted knees can represent a diagnostic challenge. An undisplaced tibial plateau or femoral condyle fracture may be deceptively pain-free; the elderly and osteoporotic patients can fracture after a relatively minor injury and delayed diagnosis is surprisingly common.

The acutely injured knee is usually too swollen and painful to assess properly in the first few days. There is a great temptation to aspirate the knee to provide pain relief. This should not really be done unless the patient is in extremis. Any pain that bad probably warrants an X-ray too. Aspirating a joint in any situation outside a theatre runs the risk of introducing an infection. The effusion or haemarthrosis will almost certainly re-collect in a day or so, and it is an excellent culture medium for the bacteria that have just been introduced. A knee effusion can be diagnostic. If the swelling comes on immediately, it suggests that something with a good blood supply has bled (ie a fractured bone or cruciate ligament). Conversely, an effusion from a torn meniscus or sprain takes a few hours to develop. Obviously, a fracture will need referral, but any haemarthrosis needs an X-ray.

Once the acute pain has settled, clinical examination of the knee is almost as accurate as magnetic resonance imaging (MRI) in terms of diagnosis.

- Commonly it is the medial collateral ligament that is sprained. This will be tender at a point about 2 cm above and below the medial femoro-tibial joint line. Valgus stressing of the knee will also be painful.

- A meniscal tear will be tender at the level of the femoro-tibial joint line, in the dip you can feel just above the medial edge of the tibial plateau. A tear will give the classic symptoms of locking and giving way.

- Anterior cruciate ligament (ACL) tears are also common. They present with a tense haemarthrosis and are usually too painful to assess properly initially. Once the pain has settled, the patient will often complain of an unstable or 'loose' knee which they have no confidence in. The anterior drawer test (see Figure 12.3) is positive. Everyone has some degree of movement with the anterior drawer test, so compare to the other knee. Remember that West Africans, Asians and others with hypermobile joints will have more movement than usual, but there should still be a firm, definite end point to the drawer. Specific ACL physiotherapy will develop the thigh musculature to give stability to the knee. Most of the time, this is enough for all but the sportiest of patients. Remember that the New Zealand All Blacks had such well developed thighs that they could win the World Cup with only three intact cruciates between the 15 of them! ACL reconstruction is becoming more commonplace, but it is a major procedure with the need to have at least 4 months of postoperative physiotherapy to get any benefit. There is currently no proof that reconstructing the ACL will stop the progression of osteoarthritis that is inevitable with an ACL-deficient knee.

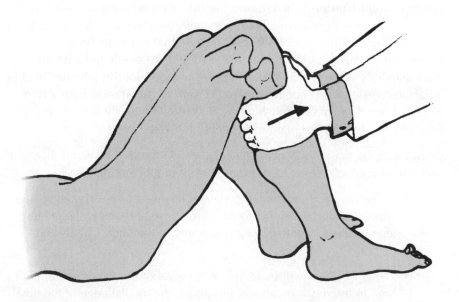

Figure 12.3 Anterior drawer test. Sit on the foot, check the hamstrings are relaxed and then try to pull the tibia gently and slowly towards you

LOCKED KNEES

Locked knees are an urgent problem. Locking is often overdiagnosed when the patient is in the acutely painful stage. A knee that does not move at all in any direction is not 'locked', but usually has a tense effusion or haemarthrosis. A true locked knee is one that can flex and extend up to a point, but cannot fully extend. The patient will often say that they have to shake or jiggle the knee in a particular way to unlock it. It results from the presence of a loose body or torn meniscus jamming the knee joint. The pressure necrosis from this jammed body leads to full-thickness cartilage loss. Arthroscopy should be carried out within a week or two, and often a referral to the Fracture Clinic is the only way to get the patient seen and operated on quickly enough.

SEPTIC ARTHRITIS

Septic arthritis is a very urgent problem. Pus in a joint will permanently dissolve all the cartilage within a day or so, and the patient will often develop fatal overwhelming sepsis a few days later unless the joint is drained. Fortunately, septic arthritis is quite rare. A patient with an established septic arthritis will not be able to weight-bear or move the affected joint at all. They will also be systemically unwell. More often the diagnosis is a rheumatological one in the adult, or a reactive synovitis in a child who has recently suffered from a coryzal-type episode.

FREQUENTLY MISSED DIAGNOSES

Most orthopaedics is common sense and there is rarely a diagnostic challenge. Usually a sprain will get better and function will recover. Sometimes though, a rarer disease presents and a delay in diagnosis and treatment will result in a poorer outcome. Most of these diagnoses are various types of avascular necrosis (AVN).

HIP

- **Perthes' disease** (avascular necrosis of the hip) in children is quite common. It is a self-limiting condition most of the time, but the patient should still be referred for follow-up, as the femoral head can end up distorted and needing either corrective surgery or a very early hip replacement. It is mainly a disease of boys aged 4–8 years. It presents with pain in the groin or with pain referred to the knee. It is an orthopaedic maxim that if you must examine or X-ray any part of a limping child, make it the pelvis, as the majority of treatable problems are sited here.

- **Slipped upper femoral epiphysis (SUFE)** is also a problem of young boys. The child is usually peripubescent (11–14 years) and is classically overweight and delayed in their sexual development. The young immature growth plates at the top of the femur are unable to stand such a weight, and they begin to literally slip off the top of the femur. This is either an acute event, or happens as an acute on chronic event. The boy will complain of groin pain, but again this is often referred to the knee. There will be a limitation in hip rotation compared with the other side (best seen when the hip is rotated while in a flexed position). An antero-posterior (AP) pelvic X-ray will often be normal, so remember to ask for a frog lateral view as well. If an acute SUFE is missed, then it cannot be reduced and the femoral head will be deformed. A chronic slip still needs fixing in situ and the normal side is usually fixed prophylactically.

- Adults are at risk of **avascular necrosis of the femoral head** too. It will present as groin or knee pain, and is more common in alcoholics, those on steroids, pregnant women, scuba divers or people with a prothrombotic tendency. It is detectable on a pelvic X-ray and, if caught in time, responds well to surgical decompression. Although many resolve spontaneously with no problem, AVN is another cause of femoral head deformity leading to very early hip replacement.

- **Trochanteric bursitis** typically results in a tender area over the greater trochanter. Always remember to palpate this area (more posterior than most people expect). An injection of lidocaine and 80 mg of methylprednisolone acetate (Depo-Medrone®) can help in diagnosis and is therapeutic; the injection can be repeated three or four times.

- **Meralgia paraesthetica** is entrapment of the lateral cutaneous nerve of the thigh as it passes under the inguinal ligament. It gives pain and paraesthesia over the anterolateral skin of the thigh, unrelated to exertion. The nerve is found 2 cm along the inguinal ligament, measuring from the anterior superior iliac spine. Nerve conduction studies are useless in investigation (the nerve is too deep), but a positive Tinel's sign, or a good response to a local anaesthetic injection suggests the diagnosis.

True hip pain is usually felt in the groin. Remember to examine the joint above and below in all orthopaedic cases; referred pain is very common.

CERVICAL RIB

Neurological or vascular problems in the arm can arise from entrapment at a number of sites. Always remember to examine the neck in a patient with hand or arm symptoms. A cervical rib can present in a variety of ways, making it a very difficult diagnosis. Any patient who has paraesthesia or pain, or the vascular symptoms of pallor or claudication in the arm should be tested for the presence of a cervical rib. Even the term itself is misleading. Although a thoracic inlet view will demonstrate a true cervical rib, only 20% of cervical ribs are actually radio-opaque; an MRI is needed to demonstrate the more usual fibrous bands. Spurling's test for a cervical rib involves standing the patient up, pulling the affected arm towards the floor with one hand and then pushing the patient's chin over towards the affected shoulder while extending their neck. This will reproduce the symptoms if a cervical rib is present.

WRIST AND HAND

- **Skier's thumb and gamekeeper's thumb** are injuries of the ulnar-sided collateral ligament between the metacarpal and proximal phalanx of the thumb. Injuries occur when the thumb is forcibly radially deviated (as when a ski pole is caught and pulled from the grip) and this can tear the ligament. Test it as if the MCPJ is a small knee – fix the metacarpal with one hand, and use your other hand to varus/valgus stress the rest of the thumb. Compare with the other side. Chronic attenuation of the ligament (from wringing the necks of birds) gives a thumb that is weak and unstable when radially deviated at the MCPJ. Both ligaments can be repaired if the symptoms warrant it.

- **Kienböck's disease** is avascular necrosis of the lunate. It presents with wrist pain, with or without tenderness over the lunate. It is one of the most important differential diagnoses of wrist pain, as it can sometimes be treated if caught early. An X-ray is diagnostic.

FOOT

- **Freiberg's disease** is avascular necrosis of the head of the second metatarsal. The patient is tender over this point and an X-ray will confirm the diagnosis. Again, early referral is indicated.

- **Morton's neuroma** is a neuroma of the digital nerve of the toes. It causes a typical pain over the midfoot and paraesthesia over the toe webs. The Mulder click is not often found, but is diagnostic; when the foot is rolled from flat to arched (as you look end on at the toes) you feel a click as the neuroma is trapped between the metatarsals. The neuroma can be excised.

- **Tibialis posterior tendon dysfunction** is quite common, considering so few people have heard of it! The usual presentation is medial foot or ankle pain. The tibialis posterior muscle tendon is prone to tenosynovitis and even rupture, leaving a painful, flat foot. To test it, sit the patient in a chair, rest the bad foot on the opposite knee with the leg in a 'figure 4' position and hold your hand just above the metatarsophalangeal (MTP) joint of the affected foot. In this position, the action of the tibialis posterior muscle is to lift the MTP joint towards the ceiling. If this movement is weak or if there is pain on resistance, tibialis posterior tenosynovitis is likely. Pain and tenderness will be felt at a point just behind the medial malleolus and walking on tiptoe will be painful. The condition can be treated with insoles, NSAIDs and physiotherapy.

- **Plantar fibromas** are often misdiagnosed as warts or ganglions. They present as a hard painful lump, usually on the medial arch. They are best treated with padded insoles, as they almost always recur after local excision.

- **Tarsal tunnel syndrome** is analogous to carpal tunnel syndrome. The medial calcaneal branch of the posterior tibial nerve supplies the skin over the medial hindfoot. It can become trapped in a tunnel an inch or so below the medial malleolus, leading to paraesthesia over the skin area that it supplies. Tinel's sign is often positive, and, as in the wrist, steroid injections or surgical release is effective.

- **Plantar fasciitis** is the most common cause of foot pain. It gives pain over the plantar aspect of the calcaneum. It is very easy to diagnose, but much harder to treat. Calcaneal spurs are often seen on X-ray, but they are incidental findings and removing them leaves a painful scar and almost never helps the underlying pain. Conservative options such as cushioning heel pads and physiotherapy (see below) are usually successful. The problem often lasts for 6 or 9 months, and is very debilitating and depressing for patient and doctor alike. Steroid injections may be given in resistant cases, but are very painful to administer, have no proof of benefit and usually need repeating.

PHYSIOTHERAPY FOR PLANTAR FASCIITIS

- Stand 1 metre from a wall. Keep the knees straight and heels on the ground and then lean into the wall, thus stretching the Achilles tendons. Hold this position for several seconds as the Achilles tendons tighten. Repeat ten times consecutively, five or six times per day.

- Sit in a chair, with the knees flexed to 90° and the feet flat on the floor. Lift the foot upwards, keeping the heel on the floor. Again, hold this position and repeat.

- Roll the arch of the foot over a tin of baked beans. This stretches and massages the plantar fascia directly.

LIMB LENGTH DISCREPANCIES

Having one leg shorter than the other is very common. It is often unrecognised and differences of up to 2 cm can easily be missed and are of no clinical significance. Many scolioses are actually the result of a short leg. This can be proved simply by seeing whether the scoliosis disappears when the patient is sitting down. Any limb length discrepancies in children warrant a referral; they should be monitored to see if the discrepancy worsens. Osteoarthritic destruction of a joint or malunion of a fracture are the commonest causes of limb shortening (eg a fractured neck of femur). In this case, as well as addressing the underlying osteoporosis, referral for a shoe raise (or asking a cobbler to provide a simple one) will often make walking easier and less painful.

BACK PAIN

Around 80% of the population can expect at least one episode of severe back pain in their lifetime. It is the presenting symptom of many other diseases. Most episodes are self-limiting and will just need simple analgesia. There are, however, some serious and some treatable conditions to keep in mind.

Spinal stenosis gives dermatomal paraesthesia and pain in the legs on exertion; this can be unilateral or bilateral. Rest relieves the pain after 10–15 minutes. Patients usually get relief by leaning forward (eg leaning onto a shopping trolley, or cycling); this opens up the space in the spine. A differential diagnosis is vascular claudication. Epidurals or surgical correction can often be remarkably beneficial, even in the unfit elderly patient.

Facet joint arthritis gives classic pain on extension (arching) of the back and tenderness over the facet joints (an inch either side of the spinous processes). The facet joints can be injected under radiographic control with local anaesthetic and steroid, although the results are rarely dramatic or permanent. Osteoporotic vertebral crush fractures hardly ever need surgery unless they are compromising the spinal cord or cauda equina. In the acute phase, bisphosphonates help greatly with pain relief. Injecting the vertebral body with bone cement can also reduce pain in resistant cases.

Prolapsed intervertebral discs are very common. Cauda equina compression should be excluded by close questioning regarding saddle paraesthesia and alteration in bowel or bladder function. Unfortunately it is never as classic as the books describe and most cases will have had only a very subtle alteration in the sensation of opening the bowels or urinating. The evidence recommends decompression as soon as possible and definitely within 48 hours from the first onset of symptoms. Most prolapsed intervertebral discs do not compress the cauda equina. The natural history of the condition is that the pain and nerve root compression will settle within 6–9 weeks. Initial treatment involves analgesia, physiotherapy and staying as active as possible. Surgery is only of use at relieving leg pain and may make back pain worse. Decompression is indicated for very severe leg pain or for leg pain that is not getting better after several months of physiotherapy.

Several non-orthopaedic diagnoses cause back pain and these need to be excluded, especially in the elderly. They include aortic aneurysm, hepatic, biliary or pancreatic pathology, renal stones or tumour, myeloma, secondary deposits (breast or prostate), osteomalacia, rheumatological disease, osteomyelitis and tuberculosis (TB). A thorough abdominal examination and blood tests including FBC, ESR, prostate-specific antigen (PSA), calcium, liver and bone profile will aid in diagnosis.

ORTHOPAEDIC MALIGNANCY

Most lumps and bumps in the limbs are benign. However, a GP can still expect to see one or two sarcomas in their career. Late diagnosis is distressingly common, and most sarcomas have been treated by a GP or non-specialist for an average of a year before diagnosis. There are a few rules to follow:

- Trauma is the most common presentation and may be misleading; patients try to remember something to explain their lump.

- Children are very often affected.

- Most tumours present around the knee.

- Abscess or haematoma are common misdiagnoses. If one of these conditions is just not getting better, then think of sarcoma.

- Do not incise or even aspirate a suspected tumour. This will seed it through the leg compartments and could make amputation inevitable.

- Tumours are hot and painful.

- Any patient with a lump larger than a golf ball should be referred.

- Ultrasound can differentiate most lumps.

OSTEOARTHRITIS

OSTEOARTHRITIS OF THE WRIST, THUMB OR FINGERS

This is almost universal in the elderly. It is not normally particularly painful, but there are surgical options available. An arthrodesis (fusion) or prosthetic replacement of the joint can provide almost full pain relief with no real loss of flexibility or function. These are simple day case procedures and should be considered if the patient is in pain.

OSTEOARTHRITIS OF THE KNEE

Osteoarthritis (OA) of the knee is very common and is usually found between the femur and tibia. In younger patients, the problem is more often in the joint between the patella and its groove on the femur. This causes the classic 'anterior knee pain', ie pain felt over the front of the patella which is made worse on squatting, climbing stairs, rising from a low chair, etc. In some patients, a maltracking patella (where the patella runs too much to one side of the groove during flexion and extension) is the underlying problem; usually the patella runs too laterally in its groove, and this can be seen during flexion. Physiotherapy aims to strengthen the medial quadriceps, thereby pulling the patella more medially.

There are several management options available to the GP for knee OA, in addition to painkillers and glucosamine:

- Injections of steroid (eg 40 mg methylprednisolone (Depo-Medrone®) with lidocaine) will settle synovitis. There is often a steroid flare, making the pain worse for a few days. When injecting a knee, the patient should have their leg extended. A medial approach is probably easiest, aiming to go deep to the patella, at an angle of about 45°. A green needle should be used. The steroid should go in without much resistance.

- Hyaluronic acid and its derivatives (eg Synvisc®) are new, expensive 'cartilage concentrates' that are said to reduce symptoms and even increase joint space. About 50% of patients will get some temporary relief, and the injections (a course of three, given weekly) can be repeated ad infinitum if necessary.

- Braces have not been proved to be beneficial in most cases, but many patients do find them helpful. Their role is best seen if there is valgus or varus malalignment; in this case, the brace is worn with the aim of re-aligning the knee and thereby pushing the force back onto the less worn parts of the knee. They are supplied by the hospital Orthotics Department.

- Walking sticks should be held in the opposite hand to whichever knee is painful. During walking, the left leg and right arm go forward together, and vice versa. This means that when the bad leg is forward, taking all the weight while the good leg swings through, the arm with the stick will be forward as well, thus sharing some of the weight through the stick. It is important that a walking stick is the correct length; the elbow should be a few degrees off full extension when the patient is standing with the stick on the floor.

- Physiotherapy and hydrotherapy will strengthen the knee and stop painful instability when the leg bears weight. Pre-arthroplasty physiotherapy will make recovery from a knee replacement quicker and easier too.

ALTERNATIVES TO KNEE REPLACEMENT

Many patients are 'too young' or 'not bad enough' for a knee replacement. There are surgical options for these people and they can still be referred.

- Arthroscopic debridement is a day case procedure that provides pain relief and increased mobility in approximately 50% of patients. This has the same success rate as placebo surgery, but it is usually offered in an attempt to ward off a much more dangerous knee replacement.

- Unicondylar replacement is another day case procedure. The medial femoral condyle and medial tibial plateau are replaced. This is only suitable for medial-sided wear, but will often provide pain relief for many years, yet still allow a standard knee replacement in the future.

- Tibial/femoral osteotomy is coming back into fashion. In these the valgus or varus knee is re-aligned so as to offload the worn (concave) part of the knee, and let the lesser-worn half of the knee take the weight. Again, many years of pain relief can be expected, and knee replacement is still almost as easy years later.

PHYSIOTHERAPY EXERCISES FOR PATIENTS POST ARTHROPLASTY

After a hip replacement certain movements can dislocate the hip. The patient will have been fully informed, but, in case they forget, they should avoid extremes of internal and external rotation and hip flexion for at least 6 months; however, normal daily activities should be fine. **The following (Figures 12.6, 12.7 and 12.8) are simple exercises to initiate pending a physiotherapy appointment if pain, weakness or stiffness recur, following a hip replacement. Likewise, the exercises in figs 12.4 and 12.5 will help restore movement to a stiff knee replacement pending a physiotherapy appointment.**

KNEE EXERCISES FOR PATIENTS POST ARTHROPLASTY

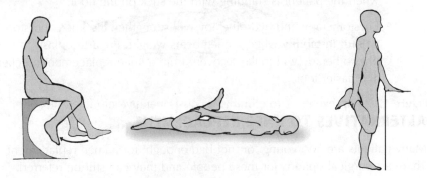

Figure 12.4 Knee exercises to increase flexion (90° is what to aim for)

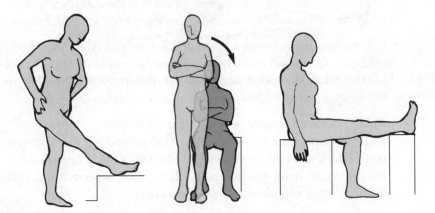

Figure 12.5 Knee exercises to regain full extension (vital to walk normally)

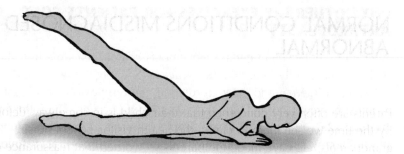

Figure 12.6 Hip exercises to strengthen hip abductors and stop Trendelenberg gait (the commonest problem)

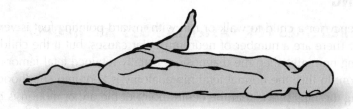

Figure 12.7 Hip exercises to eliminate a post-operative hip fixed flexion deformity.

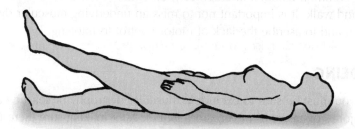

Figure 12.8 Hip exercises to increase hip flexion (beware of dislocation beyond 45°)

NORMAL CONDITIONS MISDIAGNOSED AS ABNORMAL

Parents are often very concerned that their child is in some way 'deformed'. By the time we see them in clinic, the health visitor, school nurse, grandparents, etc have made the parents so worried that reassurance can be quite difficult. The following are common problems.

INTOEING

The tendency for a child to walk or run with inward-pointing feet is very common. There are a number of neuromuscular causes, but if the child is developing normally, then the diagnosis is usually retained fetal femoral anteversion. In this, the normal fetal hip anatomy is kept into childhood. Examining the hips shows that the centre-point of the arc of motion is much more 'inwards' than normal, and so the foot will naturally come to rest in that position, especially when the child is tired. It almost always corrects before school age. Metatarsus adductus is intoeing of the big toe only and is slightly different; it sometimes needs operative correction. Clumsiness is another common complaint. Obviously, all children fall over while learning to run and walk. It is important not to miss an underlying muscular dystrophy, however, and to ascribe the lack of motor control to intoeing.

TIPTOEING

Again, you must be sure to exclude a muscular dystrophy or spastic cause. The majority of cases, however, are habitual. After making sure there is no occult spina bifida or spasticity, simple physiotherapy stretches are usually enough and tenotomy (dividing the Achilles tendon) is rarely indicated. A child who was walking normally but is now tiptoeing is much more worrying, and probably should be referred.

GENU VALGUS/VARUS

Children are born bow-legged (up to 15° is normal). By the age of 2 years the legs are usually straight. By the time children are 3 years old, 10° of knock-knees (genu valgus) is normal and this settles down to the adult shape (7° of knock-knees) by the age of 6 years. Any wide variation from this range may warrant surgical correction, and unilateral deformity is also best referred.

FLAT FEET

The foot arches are formed by the musculature of the leg. When the muscles are working hard to form an arch, they often tire and ache. This is the theory at least. In practice, flat feet are very common and not normally painful. Insoles are often given to 'help the leg muscles make an arch', but there is no real evidence of their usefulness. Surgical correction is almost unheard of for what is essentially a benign condition. As a rule of thumb, if hyperextending the big toe (Jack test) or going up on tiptoe produces some kind of arch, then nothing major is wrong.

CLICKY JOINTS

Children have relatively lax joints. Clicking in adults or children is not dangerous and does not cause arthritis in later life. Afro-Caribbean people are usually very ligamentously lax (as are Asians to a lesser degree), but you must exclude an underlying collagen disorder. Strengthening the musculature around the joint with physiotherapy can help to control the sloppy joint movements and avoid potential dislocation.

SCOLIOSIS

No one is perfectly straight. In the immature skeleton, a scoliosis can reverse, resolve or worsen before adulthood. There is very little evidence that a scoliotic spine will give any more pain as an adult than a straight spine. Also, until the deformity reaches about 100°, there is no effect on respiratory function. If an adolescent has a scoliosis of greater than 30° or 40°, the deformity is said to progress by 1° per year. It is for this reason that a very selected few adolescents with large curves have an operation.

Remember that the scoliotic deformity includes a rotational component. For this reason, it is often first noticed as a prominence of one side of the ribcage. The ribs are attached to the spine, and looking from behind as the child bends forward (Adams test) will show up the posterior rib hump and underlying scoliosis better.

OSGOOD–SCHLATTER'S

Although it is called a disease, this is almost a normal part of development. The problem is that the quadriceps pull on the immature tibial tuberosity, resulting in a chronic traction-type injury where the patella tendon insertion is painful and enlarged. It is almost inevitable if a strong athletic child puts demands on their skeleton before it is ready. It is always the overly sporty child who gets this condition and for whom the usual advice to rest (until the pain settles and for several weeks afterwards) is hardest to accept. If the patient does not rest, the pain will continue and the tibial tuberosity will be prominent in adult life.

Osgood–Schlatter's disease presents as a tender, prominent tibial tubercle.

CHONDROMALACIA PATELLAE
(LITERALLY, SOFT KNEE CARTILAGE)

This is merely a description, not a diagnosis, and presents as anterior knee pain. Occasionally, arthroscopy is needed to exclude other diagnoses, or to help plan (usually unsuccessful) patellofemoral surgery.

CHAPTER 13
PAEDIATRICS

CHAPTER 13
PAEDIATRICS

FEEDING

BREASTFEEDING

Breastfeeding is the best way to feed a baby, especially in the first few months of life. Breastfeeding 'on demand' is encouraged, but mothers should be warned that hunger is not the only reason for a child to cry, and very frequent feeds can lead to exhaustion for both the mother and baby! It is important to stimulate the breasts frequently during the early days, so that mothers are able to produce enough milk. Little and often is the best advice to give; for example, 5 minutes each side every 3 hours initially, increasing by a few minutes each day. The mother's milk will usually start to flow more readily between days 3 and 5, when about 50 ml of milk is produced per breast per feed. At this stage, the baby should be offered 15–20 minutes on the breast. There should usually be a gap of about 3 hours between feeds; if there is much less, advise the mother to offer both breasts, having fully emptied one before changing to the other, in order to avoid colic. Poor positioning is a common reason for sore nipples; the baby should be well supported, with their neck slightly extended and their mouth open wide enough to take in the whole nipple.

Cracked nipples may be helped by application of nipple shields, olive oil, damp, cold flannels, or even cold cabbage leaves between skin and bra!

Breastfed babies often produce green stool, which may be quite frequent initially, but then may only be passed once every few days.

FORMULA FEEDS

Requirements are based on the weight of the baby. In the first year, most babies need about 100 kcal/kg per day; this is equivalent to approximately 150 ml of milk per kg per day (70 ml/pound bodyweight per day), although more of the baby's calorific requirements will be made up by other food once they are weaned onto solids. Initially, the milk needs to be given in about seven to eight separate feeds, every 3 hours. However, by giving bigger feeds first thing in the morning, mid-morning and last thing at night, feeds in the middle of the night can usually be omitted by the time the baby is about 6 weeks old. Babies should gain about 180–240 g per week.

Formula feeds are based on cow's milk can be divided into three main groups:

- Whey-based (eg SMA Gold®, Aptamil®, Ostermilk® and Cow and Gate Premium®). These have a casein:whey ratio similar to that of breast milk, and are probably the most suitable for the majority of babies until they reach the age of 1 year.

- Casein-based (eg Cow and Gate Plus®, SMA White®, Milumil®). These have a higher casein:whey ratio, and are marketed for the 'hungrier' baby. However, there is little supporting evidence for their use.

- Follow-on feeds (eg SMA Progress®, Cow and Gate Step-up, Forward®). These are suitable from 6 months on, and have a higher protein, vitamin D and iron content. However, by 6 months, most babies should have started on solids, and will receive adequate nutrition from a normal formula. Follow-on feeds are only necessary if a child is failing to thrive, or has a poor diet.

After the age of 1 year, normal, full-fat cow's milk is fine. Semi-skimmed milk should not be used until the age of 2 years, and only then if the baby is receiving a well-balanced diet.

OTHER MILKS

Many mums are keen to try 'alternative' milks such as soya milks, goat's milk and sheep's milk.

- Soya milks bought in supermarkets are not suitable until the child reaches 2 years, as they are low in calories and not fully fortified with vitamins and minerals. Specially prepared soya milks are, however, available for infants, eg Wysoy®, Infasoy® and Prosobee®. These are suitable for babies with cow's milk protein intolerance, lactose intolerance, galactosaemia and for vegan babies. There is a risk that babies who are very allergic to cow's milk protein will also become allergic to soya milk. Soya milk does not protect against atopy.

- Goat's milk and sheep's milk are low in iron, vitamins A and D and folic acid. The 'Nanny' goat's milk formula is suitable for infants. There may be some cross-reactivity between mammalian proteins, so it is not suitable for children with cow's milk protein intolerance. These milks contain lactose, so there is no advantage in giving them to lactose-intolerant children.

- Enfamil AR® is a pre-thickened formula, which may help symptoms of posseting. It can only be prescribed in severe reflux disease, and only for 6 months.

- Enfamil Lacto-Free® is based on cow's milk protein, but is lactose-free, so may be useful for a short time after an episode of gastroenteritis. It should only be used in proved lactose intolerance.

SPECIALISED FORMULAS

- **Peptide-based feeds.** Examples include Pregestimil®, Nutramigen®, Pepti-Junior® and Prejomin®. These are useful for babies up to the age of 1 with cow's milk protein intolerance, lactose intolerance and galactosaemia. Pregestemil® and Pepti-Junior® can also be used for infants with malabsorption and short bowel syndrome, ie where an enteropathy has developed as a result of cow's milk protein intolerance.

- **Elemental feeds.** Examples include Neocate®, Neocate Advance®, and Elemental 028®. These are used for more severe cases of malabsorption and for short bowel syndrome.

Some experts recommend a 1–2 week trial of a peptide based feed for formula fed babies with vomiting or excessive crying. In many infants with cow's milk allergy, consideration can be given to changing to a calcium-enriched soy formula or rice milk at the age of 12 months.

MILK ALLERGIES

There are two types of 'milk allergy'. Cow's milk protein allergy (CMPA) is a true allergy, which manifests itself as severe vomiting, diarrhoea or rash when cow's milk is introduced to a breastfed baby. Options are to use a soya milk, or to prescribe a peptide-based milk (see above). Secondary CMPA can develop after an attack of gastroenteritis. Long-standing CMPA may eventually lead to an enteropathy with failure to thrive and anaemia.

Lactose intolerance is also often secondary to an attack of gastroenteritis, and is usually self-limiting. It can present with diarrhoea that occurs every time cow's milk is re-introduced. Again, treatment is to use a soya-based formula, or to prescribe a peptide-based feed. In lactose intolerance, the stool may contain more than 0.5% reducing sugars, as determined by Clinitest® tablets. Stool can also be sent to the lab to test for this.

The length of time for which a baby should stay off cow's milk is not clear. In lactose intolerance or mild secondary CMPA, 1 month to 6 weeks may be sufficient, after which cow's milk could be cautiously re-introduced at home. In true, primary CMPA, milk should be re-introduced in a hospital setting under close supervision. Mothers may need to be referred to a dietician, to be advised on how to ensure that their child still gets enough calcium.

VITAMIN SUPPLEMENTATION FOR CHILDREN

The Department of Health recommends that all children between the ages of 1 and 5 years should have vitamin supplementation with vitamins A, C and D. Formula-fed babies who take at least 500 ml of formula feed daily do not require supplementation until the age of 1 year, when most of them will stop receiving formula and go on to ordinary cow's milk. For breastfed babies whose mothers were in a good nutritional state prior to the pregnancy, supplementation may begin at 6 months. However, where there is doubt about the mother's vitamin status, additional vitamins should be given from the age of 1 month. Vitamin D levels in breast milk tend to be low, especially if the mother is herself deficient; this is common in Asian mothers. The dosage is 5 drops daily.

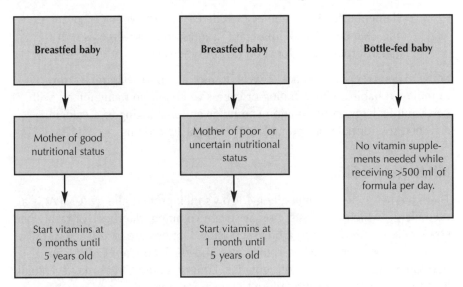

Figure 13.1 Vitamin supplementation guidance for children

Vitamins are only available free of charge for children in families receiving Income Support or an income-based Jobseeker's Allowance (under the Welfare Food Scheme). The prescription must be endorsed with 'ACBS' (Advisory Committee on Borderline Substances).

IRON DEFICIENCY

Iron deficiency is common in children; the prevalence is thought to range from 12% to 30% of 1- to 2-year-olds. Babies who are weaned late may be more at risk, for example babies who are solely breastfed beyond the age of 6 months. Iron deficiency can lead to many problems, including tiredness, increased risk of infection, impaired development and reduced IQ.

In-utero iron stores are usually depleted by the age of 6 months, and this is when children are at high risk of becoming iron-deficient. Red meat and offal are rich sources of iron. Fortified cereals and bread are other sources. Iron from meat is better absorbed than iron from cereals, pulses, eggs and green vegetables. Tannins in tea can reduce iron absorption by up to 75%.

WEANING

Weaning should usually occur between the ages of 4 months and 6 months. There is a fine balance here; in babies who are weaned too early, the kidneys and gut may not be mature enough to process solids, whereas babies who are weaned late may develop nutritional deficiencies, eg iron deficiency. By the age of 2 years, most of a child's calories should come from solids and not from milk. Weaning should begin with puréed fruit (but not berries to begin with), vegetables and non-wheat cereal. Peanuts should not usually be introduced until the age of 3 years if there is a family history of atopy. One new foodstuff should be introduced at a time.

Drinks should be offered from a cup from the age of 6 months.

By 9–12 months, the child should be eating normal, chopped-up family food.

TEETHING

Teething usually starts when the child is about 6 months old, starting with the central incisors. Children normally have their full complement of milk teeth by the age of 18–30 months. If pain is a problem, there are various teething gels that can be purchased, eg choline salicylate gel.

SMALL FONTANELLE

The size of the anterior fontanelle is variable and in some babies it does close earlier than in others. If the fontanelle seems small, the general shape of the skull should be observed; if this appears normal and the child is developing normally, it is sufficient simply to keep a check on head circumference, to ensure it is not dropping down centiles.

STICKY EYES

Sticky eyes are very common in neonates and the problem is rarely caused by serious infection.

Gonococcal conjunctivitis presents within the first 3 days of life. The baby will have a purulent discharge (often greenish in colour), with erythema of the conjunctivae, sometimes with lid swelling.

Chlamydia trachomatis either causes persistent conjunctivitis in the first week of life, again with a purulent discharge, or it presents slightly later at 7–10 days. The presentation is usually less alarming than gonococcal conjunctivitis, but a clue to the diagnosis is that it does not respond to topical chloramphenicol eye drops. With either of these conditions, swabs should be taken from the baby's eyes and the mother should have vaginal and endocervical swabs taken. Affected babies need systemic antibiotics and should be reviewed by a paediatrician.

Staphylococcal conjunctivitis sometimes occurs around days 3–5 and usually has a much milder clinical presentation than *Chlamydia* or gonococcal conjunctivitis.

If an older baby presents with persistently sticky eyes but is well in himself, the most likely cause is a partially blocked nasolacrimal duct; the duct may not open fully until the child is 3 months old. In this case, the mother should be taught to massage the lacrimal sac four times a day, in order to empty its contents. Topical antibiotics are sometimes needed, but surgery is rarely indicated unless symptoms persist beyond the age of 6 months.

RASHES

RASHES DEVELOPING IN THE FIRST WEEK

- **Erythema toxicum (neonatal urticaria):** affects about 30% of term babies. It usually starts around day 2 or day 3 and disappears in the first couple of weeks of life, with the baby remaining well throughout. The baby develops characteristic red blotches, sometimes with white pustules in the middle, often with sparing of the palms and soles. The rash is usually most prominent on the trunk and proximal limbs.

- **Milia** are small, keratin filled cysts, appearing as white papules on the face. They are often very transient, and individual lesions can disappear in a matter of hours. They can present throughout infancy.

- **Neonatal pustular melanosis** occurs in about 5% of infants, and is more common in Black male babies. The lesions are usually present at birth on the trunk and appear as small pustules that eventually crust over; the crust then peels off, leaving a red mark.

- **Miliaria**: small vesicles appearing on the baby's forehead in the first or second week of life. They are more common in hot climates because they are caused by blocked sweat ducts. They can be treated by towel drying the skin after bathing. They usually only last for a few days.

RASHES THAT APPEAR LATER

- **Baby acne** can affect up to 20% of babies, usually appearing at 3–4 weeks. It is commonly found on the face (especially the cheeks, forehead and chin), manifesting as papules, pustules and whiteheads. It usually clears up by the time the baby is about 4 months old.

BIRTHMARKS

- **Stork mark (capillary haemangioma)**: usually on the back of the neck or face, fading with time.

- **Strawberry naevus (cavernous haemangioma)**: these lesions usually develop at around 4–6 weeks of age, increase in size for the first 6 months, and then start to fade, until they are completely gone by the age of 7 years.

- **Port wine stain (capillary naevus)**: this usually occurs on the face and is a permanent birthmark.

- **Mongolian blue spot**: extremely common in non-Caucasian babies (incidence up to 90%), usually on the lower back. They fade with time, and may no longer be visible by the age of 2 years.

UNDESCENDED TESTICLES

It is usual for the testes to descend at 36 weeks of gestation, so newborn male babies should not have undescended testicles (although this is more common in premature babies). Examination of the testicles should be performed at the 6-week check and referral considered if they are not palpable in the scrotum. Descent never occurs after the age of 1 year and malignant change is 30 times more likely in the affected testicle. Sperm production is irreversibly impaired if the testis is not fixed by the age of 6 years. Most surgeons will perform orchidopexy when the child is about 4 years old. Hernias are commonly found in babies with undescended testes. If there is bilateral maldescent, consider referring the baby for karyotyping to confirm gender.

CIRCUMCISION

See Chapter 17, Urology.

BEHAVIOURAL PROBLEMS

SLEEPLESS NIGHTS

This can be an issue for both parent and child! In general, it is useful to establish whether there is any underlying cause, for example a physical problem such as eczema, asthma or reflux that keeps the child awake. If there does not appear to be any physical cause, behavioural techniques can often help. It is also useful to advise the parents to make a few environmental changes, for example ensuring the nursery is not too hot or cold, and that it is completely dark; full-length curtains lined with black-out fabric can be useful. It is important to establish a night-time routine (with bathing, nappy changing, feeding, etc), which should be followed at roughly the same time every day, ideally with the child in his or her own bedroom. The frequency and duration of daytime sleeps should be reduced. If the baby wakes every morning because of a dirty nappy, it might be worth adjusting the diet, so that the main meal is taken at lunchtime, and most of the fruit by early afternoon. Night-time feeding should be done as quickly as possible, in a darkened room, with minimal eye contact and talking. Some babies sleep better in lightweight sleeping bags.

If none of these measures seem to work, it is worth advising the parents to use a so-called 'controlled crying' technique. When the child wakes, the parent should be advised to settle them, but not talk to them or cuddle them, then to leave the room. The parents should gradually leave the child to cry for longer and longer periods before coming in to their room. There shouldn't be any exceptions, as inconsistent behaviour from the parents might make the situation worse.

PERSISTENT CRYING

Excessive crying is defined as crying for more than 3 hours a day on at least 3 days of the week, for a period of at least 3 weeks.

- It is worth trying to establish whether there is a pattern to the crying, eg if it is because the baby is hungry or too hot.

- Crying because of colic is more likely to occur in the early evening.

- It is also worth checking for any physical problems, such as eczema, oral thrush, constipation (possibly with small anal fissures around the anal margin), blocked nose, reflux, etc.

- Check that the baby is putting on weight satisfactorily and is developing normally.

- A detailed feeding history should be taken; it is possible that the mother is overfeeding her baby or that weaning has taken place too soon. The baby might be gulping air with its feeds and may need to be winded more frequently. This can occur if the hole in the teat of the baby's bottle is too small.

- Check the mother for postnatal depression (see Chapter 14, Psychiatry, for the Edinburgh Postnatal Depression Scale).

FOOD REFUSAL

This is common in toddlers, often as a way of asserting their independence. If a child is gaining weight satisfactorily, then parents should be advised to adopt a 'take it or leave it' attitude. They should never confront the child about food, but leave the food out and allow the child to help him- or herself.

FOOD INTOLERANCE

Food intolerance is becoming an increasingly common diagnosis, although true IgE-mediated allergy is rare. Most true food allergies occur in children and 93% occur in response to only the following eight foods:

- Egg
- Peanuts
- Milk
- Soy
- Tree nuts, eg pecans
- Shellfish
- Fish
- Wheat.

When certain foods are suspected of causing a reaction, they should be eliminated from the child's diet, under the supervision of a dietician. Most children grow out of their intolerances to wheat, milk, egg and soy, often before the age of 3 years. However, allergies to peanuts, shellfish, tree nuts and fish are often lifelong. Skin-prick testing with food extracts can be done for children who are suspected of having a true IgE-mediated food allergy. This is only useful in diagnosing IgE allergy; it is not very useful in food 'intolerance'.

NOCTURNAL ENURESIS

THE NUMBER OF CHILDREN WHO REGULARLY WET THE BED

- 1 in 6 five-year-olds

- 1 in 7 seven-year-olds

- 1 in 20 ten-year-olds

- 1 in 50–100 teenagers

USEFUL CONTACT INFORMATION

ERIC (Enuresis Resource and Information Centre). tel: 0117 9603060, www.eric.org.uk – free, confidential advice can be given, and parents can also purchase enuresis alarms and literature.

USEFUL ADVICE

Parents should begin toilet training at the age of 2 years. The child should always be praised for correct behaviour, but not punished for having an accident.

Enuresis can be primary or secondary (if the child was dry for at least 6 months before the wetting started). Common causes of secondary enuresis include emotional upset, eg parents separating (ask about other behavioural problems at school or home), diet (eg consuming an inappropriately high quantity of fluid, especially before bedtime), constipation, diabetes and urinary tract infection (UTI). A urine sample should be checked for glucose and sent for culture. The child should also be examined for any signs of occult spinal problems.

If no organic cause is found, various behavioural methods could be tried:

- Reducing quantity of fluid consumed from 2 hours before bedtime.

- Star charts are especially helpful in the over-5s. They should be used to reward behaviour that the child can control, eg getting out of bed to use the toilet during the night. They are thought to be effective in about 20% of cases.

- Enuresis alarms. These work by using a pad system, which, when wet, activates the alarm. Alarms are available to wear either inside the child's underwear (costing approximately £50–£70), or in the bed (at a cost of £100–£115). The objective is for the child to stop urinating when the alarm goes off. A systematic review (*Cochrane Review; Cochrane Library*, Issue 2, 2004) found that 45% of children using the alarms stay dry after treatment has finished, and about 66% stay dry while they use the alarm. Body-worn alarms are probably more effective than bed alarms. It is unlikely that a child under 5 years old will be able to use the alarm successfully.

- Alarms plus behavioural programmes; for example, the child is asked to deliberately delay micturition during the day, to increase functional bladder capacity. Waking the child to go to the toilet when the alarm sounds, and changing their sheets straight away can be helpful but is very difficult to manage in practice.

Medications that can be tried include desmopressin and imipramine. Desmopressin is an analogue of antidiuretic hormone (ADH), and reduces urine volume. It is available as a tablet or as a nasal spray, to be taken just before going to bed, and is licensed for children of 5 years and older. Potential adverse effects include hyponatraemia as a result of fluid overload; the child should therefore be 'fluid-restricted' for 1 hour before and until 8 hours after administration. Imipramine is a tricyclic antidepressant and is licensed for enuresis in children from the age of 6 years. It is potentially fatal in overdose and should only be initiated by a specialist team.

COMMON VIRAL RASHES IN CHILDHOOD

ROSEOLA INFANTUM (EXANTHEMA SUBITUM)

This is caused by human herpesvirus 6 and is very common in babies aged between 6 and 18 months; most children have been infected by the age of 2 years. The incubation period is 5–15 days and it presents with fever (lasting 3–5 days on average) and a maculopapular rash over the face, neck and trunk, which usually appears as the fever subsides.

FIFTH DISEASE (SLAPPED CHEEK DISEASE)

This is caused by parvovirus B19 (see also Chapter 10, Obstetrics). The peak incidence is between 5 and 10 years of age. There is an incubation period of 7–17 days and children usually present initially with symptoms of headache and malaise, followed by an asymptomatic period of about a week before the characteristic rash develops. This often begins on the face (typical slapped cheek appearance), then spreads to the trunk and limbs, where it has a fine maculopapular appearance.

HAND, FOOT AND MOUTH DISEASE

The peak age of incidence is between 10 months and 3 years, and it is caused by coxsackievirus A16, A19 and enterovirus 71. The incubation period is 3–7 days and it presents with fever, malaise and headache, followed by pharyngitis and vesicular lesions on the palms of the hands, soles of the feet, on the buttocks, genitals and in the mouth.

CHICKENPOX

The incubation period is 10–21 days and children are infectious from 48 hours before the rash appears until the time when the vesicles crust over. (See also Chapter 10, Obstetrics)

MEASLES

The incubation period is 7–21 days and there are often prodromal symptoms of cough, coryza and conjunctivitis. Koplik's spots (typically, small white lesions) can sometimes be seen on the buccal mucosa, and associated otitis media is common. The rash usually starts behind the ears and then spreads over the trunk.

RUBELLA

The incubation period is 14–21 days. The rash is maculopapular and starts on the face, and then spreads to the trunk and extremities. There is often associated posterior cervical lymphadenopathy. The patient is infective from 5 days before until 5 days after the rash appears.

CHILDHOOD MIGRAINE

The prevalence of childhood migraine is thought to be as high as 10%, and it is the most common cause of severe, recurrent headache in children. The headache is typically bilateral and lasts for between 1 and 72 hours. There is often associated photophobia or phonophobia. The natural history of the condition is poorly understood, although it appears that up to 50% of patients continue to suffer from migraines into adulthood. Abdominal migraine is a separate condition in which the child complains of central abdominal pain lasting 1–72 hours, associated with nausea, vomiting and anorexia.

TREATMENT

- Self-help measures, eg keeping a symptom diary to discover any possible triggers, such as particular foods, stress, lack of sleep.

- Analgesics: these should be taken early on in the course of the headache. In order to reduce the risk of medication-overuse headache, analgesia should ideally not be used for more than 2 days per week. The two drugs most commonly prescribed are paracetamol and ibuprofen; opioids are not recommended. It may help the situation if the school is informed, so that the child is able to take their medication as soon as the headache starts. Rectal preparations of paracetamol can be useful if there is concomitant nausea or vomiting.

- Triptans: sumatriptan, given as a nasal spray, is licensed for use in adolescents aged between 12 and 17 years, but should be initiated by a specialist.

- Anti-emetics: domperidone is licensed for relief of nausea and vomiting in children, at doses of 0.25–0.5mg/kg tds or qds. Prochlorperazine (Stemetil®, possibly given rectally) or an antihistamine are other options. Metoclopramide is not recommended because of the risk of acute dystonic reactions.

- Prophylaxis can be considered in children who have migraines more frequently than twice a month or whose migraines are very severe, causing them to miss school. Propranolol is likely to be the drug of choice in this case. There is limited evidence that the herbal remedy feverfew may help to reduce the frequency and severity of migraine. However, there are very few trials involving children.

CHAPTER 14
PSYCHIATRY AND SUBSTANCE MISUSE

BENZODIAZEPINES

Benzodiazepines are addictive, whether used at normal or high doses. The Committee on Safety of Medicines (CSM) recommend that they should only be used for a period of 2-4 weeks, and only then for severe anxiety or insomnia. Approximately 35% of patients who use them continuously for 6 months experience withdrawal symptoms when treatment is stopped. A minority of patients experience these effects after only a few weeks of use. Short-acting benzodiazepines such as lorazepam and alprazolam are more difficult to stop than long-acting medications such as diazepam or chlordiazepoxide and patients on short-acting drugs are more likely to experience serious withdrawal phenomena, such as convulsions. There are several problems associated with the long-term use of benzodiazepines, including confusion, memory loss, ataxia, dysarthria and a 50% increased risk of traffic accidents, according to one study (American Journal of Psychiatry 2001, 158: 625-55).

WITHDRAWAL SYMPTOMS

Symptoms can be both psychological and physical. The convulsions can sometimes occur, particularly in patients who have been taking a benzodiazepine for a prolonged period. Commonly encountered symptoms include:

- Acute anxiety or psychosis
- Insomnia
- Paranoia
- Loss of appetite
- Depression

CHAPTER 14
PSYCHIATRY AND SUBSTANCE MISUSE

BENZODIAZEPINES

Benzodiazepines are addictive, whether used at normal or high doses. The Committee on Safety of Medicines (CSM) recommends that they should only be used for a period of 2–4 weeks, and only then for acute, severe anxiety or insomnia. Approximately 33% of patients who use them continuously for 6 months experience withdrawal symptoms when treatment is stopped. A minority of patients experience these effects after only a few weeks of use. Short-acting benzodiazepines such as lorazepam and alprazolam are more difficult to stop than long-acting medications such as diazepam or chlordiazepoxide and patients on short-acting drugs are more likely to experience serious withdrawal phenomena such as convulsions. There are several problems associated with the long-term use of benzodiazepines, including confusion, memory loss, ataxia, dysarthria and a 50% increased rate of hip fracture in the elderly, according to one study (*American Journal of Psychiatry* 2001; **158**: 892–898).

WITHDRAWAL SYMPTOMS

Symptoms can be both psychological and physical. Convulsions can sometimes occur, particularly in patients who have been taking benzodiazepines for a prolonged period. Commonly encountered symptoms include:

- **Acute anxiety or psychosis**
- **Insomnia**
- **Paranoia**
- **Loss of appetite**
- **Depression**

- Panic attacks

- Hyperactivity

- Depersonalisation/derealisation

- Anger/irritability

- Ataxia, tremor, twitching, double vision

- Convulsions

- Abdominal pain and diarrhoea.

These symptoms commonly start 3–7 days after the benzodiazepines are stopped, and are often quite marked initially, but may persist in a milder form for several weeks; however, the effects are usually less severe after the first couple of weeks. Most patients are almost back to normal after about 1 month, but may suffer from minor symptoms for several months.

METHODS OF WITHDRAWAL

It is usually possible to withdraw from benzodiazepines in the community, but, occasionally, inpatient treatment may be required, particularly if the patient has a tendency to seizures, if there has been prolonged usage or if they are very frail and elderly.

Withdrawal usually takes place over about 4–20 weeks (or sometimes even longer). The patient needs to understand that close supervision will be necessary and that they will need to attend surgery regularly.

1   Agree a 'contract' with the patient, for example that they will come to the surgery once a week for their prescription, and the period over which withdrawal is to take place is fixed.

2   Change the patient over to a longer-acting benzodiazepine (usually diazepam), to be taken at night. For equivalent dosages, see Table 14.1.

3   Reduce the dose of diazepam slowly, eg at a rate of 2 mg/week or 2 mg per fortnight. If the patient experiences withdrawal symptoms, do not reduce the dose further until these symptoms abate.

4   Watch out for other problems, such as increasing use of alcohol, cigarettes and the emergence of depressive symptoms.

Drug	Dose that is equivalent to 5 mg diazepam (in mg)
Alprazolam	0.5
Lorazepam	0.5
Loprazolam	0.5
Nitrazepam	5
Flurazepam (Dalmane®)	7.5
Temazepam	10
Chlordiazepoxide	15

Table 14.1: Equivalent doses for long-acting benzodiazepines

ALCOHOL

Problem drinking is very common in the UK. It is thought that about 30% of divorces and 40% of domestic violence cases are directly attributable to alcohol. The UK recommended limits are 14 units per week for women and 21 units for men. Consumption of >3 units per day for women or >5 units per day for men is thought to be hazardous. Problem drinking and alcohol dependency may result in the patient's driving license being revoked – see Chapter 3, DVLA regulations.

WHAT IS A UNIT?

One unit of alcohol in the UK is defined as a drink containing 8 g of ethanol. This is equivalent to:

- Half a pint of average-strength beer, lager, or cider (3–4% alcohol by volume)
- A small pub measure (25 ml) of spirits (40% alcohol by volume)
- A standard pub measure (50 ml) of fortified wine, eg sherry, port (20% alcohol by volume).

A small glass (125 ml) of average-strength wine (12% alcohol by volume) contains 1.5 units of alcohol. Therefore, there are 9 units in a bottle of wine.

A standard pub measure (35 ml) of spirits (40% alcohol by volume) contains 1.5 units of alcohol. A 750-ml bottle of spirits contains 30 units.

WHAT IS THE BEST WAY TO ASSESS WHETHER A PATIENT IS SHOWING SIGNS OF PROBLEM DRINKING?

The Alcohol Use Disorders Identification Test (the AUDIT questionnaire) (Table 14. 2) was developed by the WHO as a screening tool to detect problem drinking, and is designed to be used in a primary care setting. It is more accurate than the traditional CAGE questionnaire, being at least 92% sensitive and 93% specific. It consists of ten questions, which take about 2 minutes to complete.

The scores are indicated in brackets next to the answers. A score of 8 or more in men and 7 or more in women indicates a strong probability of hazardous or harmful alcohol consumption. A score of 13 or more is indicative of significant alcohol-related harm/dependence; these patients should be advised to abstain completely from alcohol.

AUDIT QUESTIONNAIRE*

Please RING your answer to each of the 10 questions.

1 How often do you have a drink containing alcohol?

(0) Never   (1) Monthly or less   (2) Two to four times a month
(3) Two or three times a week   (4) Four or more times a week

2 How many drinks containing alcohol do you have on a typical day when you are drinking?

(0) 1 or 2   (1) 3 or 4   (2) 5 or 6   (3) 7 to 9
(4) 10 or more

3 How often do you have six or more drinks on one occasion?

(0) Never   (1) Less than monthly   (2) Monthly   (3) Weekly
(4) Daily or almost daily

4 How often during the past year have you found that you were not able to stop drinking once you had started?

(0) Never   (1) Less than monthly   (2) Monthly   (3) Weekly
(4) Daily or almost daily

5 How often during the past year have you failed to do what was normally expected of you because of drinking?

(0) Never   (1) Less than monthly   (2) Monthly   (3) Weekly
(4) Daily or almost daily

6 How often during the past year have you needed a first drink in the morning to get yourself going after a heavy drinking session?

(0) Never   (1) Less than monthly   (2) Monthly   (3) Weekly
(4) Daily or almost daily

7 How often during the past year have you had a feeling of guilt or remorse after drinking?

(0) Never   (1) Less than monthly   (2) Monthly   (3) Weekly
(4) Daily or almost daily

8 How often during the past year have you been unable to remember what happened the night before because you had been drinking?

(0) Never   (1) Less than monthly   (2) Monthly   (3) Weekly
(4) Daily or almost daily

* with copyright permission from WHO; *The Alcohol Use Disorder Identification Test: Guidelines for Use in Primary Care*, 2nd Edition, WHO, 2001, p.18.

9 Have you or has someone else been injured as a result of your drinking?

(0) No   (2) Yes, but not in the past year   (4) Yes, during the past year

10 Has a relative or friend or a doctor or other health worker been concerned about your drinking or suggested you cut down?

(0) No   (2) Yes, but not in the past year   (4) Yes, during the past year

Table 14.2: The Alcohol Use Disorders Identification Test (the AUDIT questionnaire)

WITHDRAWING FROM ALCOHOL IN THE COMMUNITY

Most patients are able to withdraw from alcohol in the community. Exceptions are patients who have had a history of delirium tremens (or other complications) after previous attempts at withdrawal, epileptic patients, patients with significant psychiatric disease, drug users, people with a long history of extreme alcohol abuse, people who live alone and have no social support, patients who are confused and those with significant co-morbidity.

Benzodiazepines can be used in primary care for patients who would like to stop drinking, but who suffer from withdrawal symptoms when they try. They are rarely needed for men who drink less than 15 units per day or women who drink less than 10 units. They should be used for a maximum period of 7 days (Scottish Intercollegiate Guidelines Network (SIGN) 2003) and only on the clear understanding that the patient will stop drinking altogether before starting the withdrawal regime. Benzodiazepines reduce the signs and symptoms of alcohol withdrawal and the risk of seizures or delirium tremens, and they are currently considered the drugs of choice in the treatment of acute alcohol detoxification. Chlordiazepoxide is the preferred benzodiazepine for people managed in the community, because it has a slower onset of action than diazepam and therefore has less potential for abuse. Diazepam has similar efficacy to chlordiazepoxide but has greater potential for abuse; patients who are given a prescription for it should therefore be monitored closely. Clomethiazole should not be used in alcohol detoxification in primary care, due to the risk of respiratory depression in combination with alcohol, and the danger of dependence (SIGN 2003).

Delirium tremens is a potentially life-threatening condition which starts 48–72 hours after the patient stops drinking. It is marked by agitation, confusion, paranoia and hallucinations. The patient is at risk of seizures, hyperthermia, dehydration, electrolyte imbalance, shock and chest infection, and should be referred urgently to hospital.

WITHDRAWAL REGIME

In general, chlordiazepoxide will be needed for 7 days, during which time the dose will be tapered off as described in Table 14.3. It should ideally be dispensed daily, with the patient coming to the surgery so that compliance can be assessed; if they smell of alcohol or admit to drinking, the chlordiazepoxide should be stopped. Doses should probably be halved in elderly patients.

Day	Chlordiazepoxide dose (mg)			
	On waking	12 noon	6 pm	Bedtime
1	20–30	20–30	20–30	20–30
2	20–30	20–30	20–30	20–30
3	15	15	15	15
4	15	15	15	15
5	10	10	10	10
6	10	–	–	10
7	–	–	–	10

Table 14.3: Dosing schedule for chlordiazepoxide in the withdrawal regime

Most patients will need additional support from friends and family and also from the various voluntary organisations that exist in the UK (see Useful Contact Information, p. 329), such as Alcoholics Anonymous (AA), Women for Sobriety and Secular Organisations for Sobriety. Al-Anon helps relatives, friends and colleagues of problem drinkers; and Al-Teen helps young people who have a parent, relative, or friend with an alcohol problem.

If the GP decides to monitor a patient's bloods while they withdraw from alcohol, it is worth noting that gamma-glutamyl transferase (GGT) usually returns to normal in a few weeks (unless there is significant liver damage), but the mean cell volume (MCV) may take several months to normalise.

VITAMIN B SUPPLEMENTATION IN ALCOHOL DEPENDENCY

People with chronic alcohol dependence are often malnourished and deficient in vitamins, especially thiamine (vitamin B1), usually because of reduced absorption. The SIGN guideline recommends that people who have a chronic alcohol problem and whose diet may be deficient should be given oral thiamine indefinitely. The *British National Formulary* recommended doses are:

Severe deficiency: 200–300 mg per day. This should be given in divided doses to maximise absorption.

Mild chronic deficiency: 10–25 mg per day.

VITAMIN B SUPPLEMENTS DURING DETOXIFICATION

Detoxification may precipitate Wernicke's encephalopathy, which must be treated urgently with parenteral thiamine. Signs of possible Wernicke–Korsakoff syndrome (which may progress to encephalopathy) in someone undergoing detoxification include confusion, ataxia, ophthalmoplegia, nystagmus, memory disturbance, hypothermia, hypotension and coma.

- Anyone undergoing alcohol detoxification at home should be given oral thiamine (200 mg daily) for 5–7 days (*Drugs and Therapeutics Bulletin*, 2003; 41(7): 49–50).

People who are severely malnourished or who have long-standing dependence are at highest risk of developing Wernicke–Korsakoff syndrome during alcohol withdrawal. There is a strong argument for admitting such high-risk people to hospital during detoxification for intravenous administration of vitamin supplements (Pabrinex®).

Guidelines from the European Society for Parenteral and Enteral Nutrition recommend that patients with chronic liver disease and inadequate food intake are given 35–40 kcal/kg/day of non-protein energy with 1.5g/kg/day of protein.

ANTIDEPRESSANTS

A useful initial screening tool to use in general practice consists of the following two questions:

- 'Have you felt down, depressed or hopeless very often in the past month?'

- 'Have you found that you have taken little interest or pleasure in doing things in the past month?'

It has been found that 97% of people with significant depression will answer in the affirmative to at least one of these two questions. In this case, to clarify whether there is true clinical depression, it is worth using the DSM IV (*Diagnostic and Statistical Manual of Mental Disorders*, 4th edition) criteria for major depression, which are listed below:

DSM IV CRITERIA

Over the past 2 weeks, five of the following nine features should be present, of which one or more should be:

- depressed mood

- anhedonia

and then three or four of the following, to make a total of at least five:

- change in weight or appetite

- change in sleep

- agitation or retardation

- loss of energy/fatigue

- guilt/worthlessness

- poor concentration

- recurrent thoughts of death/suicide.

Many patients in general practice have so-called 'mild depression', which does not fulfil the DSM criteria; these patients are less likely to be helped by drugs, and may be better suited to psychological treatments. Self-help cognitive behavioural therapy (CBT) techniques are available on the 'mood gym' website (www.moodgym.anu.edu.au) .An excellent self-help book is *Mind over Mood* by Dennis Greenberger and Christine Padesky (Guilford Press, 1995). NICE does not recommend antidepressant treatment for mild depression in its 2004 guidelines.

CHOICE OF ANTIDEPRESSANT

Fluoxetine is not usually a good choice in the elderly, as it tends to cause agitation and anxiety. Interestingly, it is sometimes used as a drug of abuse, since it prolongs the effect of Ecstasy (although this is not usually a problem in the elderly!). Many psychiatrists favour the serotonin and noradrenaline reuptake inhibitors (SNRIs), which have a broadly similar range of action to the tricyclic antidepressants (TCAs). Venlafaxine and mirtazapine are the drugs currently available in this group, the latter being especially good for patients with insomnia. These drugs are generally more expensive than selective serotonin reuptake inhibitors (SSRIs) or TCAs, and are usually second-line agents (it is recommended that venlafaxine should only be initiated by a psychiatrist or by a GP with a specialist interest in psychiatry). If SNRIs fail to work, there are not many therapeutic options left; this is because SNRIs have all the effect of SSRIs as well as an additional effect of their own.

DURATION OF TREATMENT

Antidepressants should be used for at least 6 months after symptoms improve, and may be needed long-term for patients with recurrent major depression; for example for 2 years following a particularly severe depressive episode or in patients who have had two or more moderate or severe depressive episodes in the recent past (NICE 2004).

ST JOHN'S WORT (HYPERICUM EXTRACT W55570)

A recent RCT (*BMJ* 2005; 330: 503–5) found St John's Wort to be at least as effective as paroxetine when given in doses of 300 mg tds over 6 weeks.

SIDE-EFFECTS

TCAs and SSRIs are probably of equivalent efficacy, but SSRIs are usually better tolerated; recent NICE guidelines have recommended SSRIs as first-line treatment for depression for this reason. There has recently been concern that certain tricyclics (eg dothiepin) increase coronary heart disease (CHD) rates and are cardiotoxic. Newer TCAs such as lofepramine are probably safer in this regard.

There is also evidence that SSRIs increase the risk of gastrointestinal bleeding, probably about as much as NSAIDs or aspirin (*Drugs and Therapeutics Bulletin* 2004; 42(3): 17–18). Fluoxetine, sertraline and paroxetine are more likely to cause a bleed than other drugs in this group, but there is a relative risk of abnormal bleeding of 1.9 even with the other SSRIs (*Archives of Internal Medicine* 2004; **164**: 2367–2370). These drugs should therefore be used with caution in patients over the age of 80 and in those taking regular NSAIDs or aspirin.

SSRIs are safer than TCAs in overdose and are therefore preferred if a patient is thought to be suicidal. Certain SSRIs (eg citalopram, fluoxetine and paroxetine) are also safer in patients who still drink alcohol.

The use of SSRIs in children under the age of 18 years is controversial. Although NICE has sanctioned the use of fluoxetine (with sertraline and citalopram as second-line alternatives), the European Medicines Agency claims that no SSRI should be prescribed for children or adolescents due to concerns about increased suicide risk. Antidepressant treatment in the under-18s should not be initiated in primary care.

STOPPING ANTIDEPRESSANT TREATMENT

Antidepressants should usually be tapered off over a period of 4 weeks unless they have been used for less than 6 weeks, in which case it is safe to stop them after 1–2 weeks. Patients who have been on long-term medication may need to stop treatment even more slowly, for example by 25% of the treatment dose every 4–6 weeks (*Drugs and Therapeutics Bulletin* 1999; **37**(7): 49–52). Fluoxetine is the only antidepressant that can be stopped abruptly, unless it has been used at a dose of greater than 20 mg, when it should be reduced over 2 weeks.

The 2003 Maudsley Guidelines recommend that most antidepressants can be stopped over 4 weeks. Exceptions are paroxetine and venlafaxine, which may need to be withdrawn over 1–3 months.

CHANGING ANTIDEPRESSANTS

In general, an antidepressant should be tried for 6 weeks before deciding that it is not beneficial. If there is a partial response after a month, then the drug dosage should be increased. However, if there is no improvement after 6 weeks, the doctor may wish to change over to a new treatment. In general, there is not much therapeutic benefit to be gained from switching to another agent from the same group. Nor is there generally much point in changing from an SNRI to an SSRI. When changing antidepressant, often a strategy of 'cross-tapering' is used where the first drug is slowly reduced, while the new one is gradually introduced (Tables 14.4, 14.5). The length of time over which cross-tapering should take place is not fixed, and largely depends on the individual patient. Patients need very close supervision when changing over from one antidepressant to another.

Cross-tapering is not always necessary, for example when switching from one SSRI to another, it is often possible to make a direct swap (except when changing from fluoxetine); the effects of the second SSRI are often similar enough to the first to prevent withdrawal reactions.

	Week 1	Week 2	Week 3	Week 4
Stopping dothiepin 150 mg	100 mg od dothiepin	50 mg od dothiepin	25 mg od dothiepin	Nil
Introducing citalopram	10 mg od citalopram	10 mg od citalopram	20 mg od citalopram	20 mg od citalopram

Table 14.4: Cross-tapering: an example of changing from dothiepin to citalopram

There are potential dangers in administering two different antidepressants at the same time: some SSRIs increase the plasma concentration of tricyclics, leading to possible toxicity. If two SSRIs are given simultaneously, or a new SSRI is introduced within 4 days of stopping fluoxetine, there is a risk of serotonin syndrome. This is potentially life-threatening and features include restlessness, excess sweating, tremor, confusion, convulsions and, occasionally, death. Such patients should be admitted urgently to hospital.

Table 14.5: Advice on changing antidepressant medications (with copyright permission from The Maudsley Prescribing Guidelines 2003; Taylor & Francis Books Ltd.)

Changing from:	Changing to:					
	Tricyclics	Citalopram	Fluoxetine	Mirtazapine	Sertraline	Venlafaxine
Tricyclics (except clomipramine which should be withdrawn before starting an SSRI)	Cross-taper cautiously	Halve the dose of the tricyclic, then add citalopram, gradually tapering off dose of tricyclic	Halve the dose of the tricyclic, then add fluoxetine. Slowly withdraw the tricyclic	Cross-taper cautiously	Halve dose of tricyclic, then add sertraline, slowly withdrawing the tricyclic	Cross-taper cautiously, starting with 37.5 mg/day venlafaxine
Citalopram	Cross-taper cautiously		Stop citalopram, then start fluoxetine at 10 mg per day	Cross-taper cautiously	Stop citalopram, then start sertraline at 25 mg per day	Stop citalopram, then start venlafaxine at 37.5 mg per day. Increase very slowly
Fluoxetine	Stop fluoxetine altogether. Start tricyclic at very low dose and gradually increase	Stop fluoxetine. Wait 4–7 days, then start citalopram at 10 mg per day and increase slowly		Stop fluoxetine. Start mirtazapine cautiously	Stop fluoxetine. Wait 4–7 days, then start sertraline at 25 mg per day and increase slowly	Stop fluoxetine. Wait 4–7 days, then start venlafaxine at 37.5 mg per day, increasing slowly

Table 14.5: continued

Changing from:	Changing to:					
	Tricyclics	**Citalopram**	**Fluoxetine**	**Mirtazapine**	**Sertraline**	**Venlafaxine**
Mirtazapine	Stop mirtazapine and then start tricyclic	Stop mirtazapine, then start citalopram	Stop mirtazapine, then start fluoxetine		Stop mirtazapine, then start sertraline	Stop mirtazapine, then start venlafaxine
Sertraline	Cross-taper cautiously with very low dose of tricyclic	Withdraw sertraline first, then start citalopram	Withdraw sertraline first, then start fluoxetine	Cross-taper cautiously		Withdraw sertraline then start venlafaxine, at 37.5 mg per day, increasing very slowly
Venlafaxine	Cross-taper cautiously, starting with very low dose of tricyclic	Cross-taper cautiously, starting with citalopram 10 mg per day	Cross-taper cautiously, starting with fluoxetine 20 mg every other day	Cross-taper cautiously	Cross-taper cautiously, starting with 25 mg per day	

DEPRESSION IN THE ELDERLY

This is a common and often overlooked problem. Patients who are socially isolated, who have cognitive impairment or who have chronic disease are particularly vulnerable. The Geriatric Depression Scale (GDS) is a suitable screening test for determining the presence and severity of depression. Each 'depressive' answer scores 1 point:

1 Are you basically satisfied with your life?

2 Have you dropped many of your activities and interests?

3 Do you feel happy most of the time?

4 Do you prefer to stay at home rather than going out and doing new things?

If none of the above responses suggest depression, no further questions need to be asked.

5 Do you feel that life is empty?

6 Do you get bored often?

7 Are you in good spirits most of the time?

8 Are you afraid that something bad is going to happen to you?

9 Do you feel helpless?

10 Do you feel that you have more problems with your memory than most people?

11 Do you think it's wonderful to be alive?

12 Do you feel worthless the way you are now?

13 Do you think that most people are better off than you are?

14 Do you feel that your situation is hopeless?

15 Do you feel full of energy?

A score of 0–4 indicates that the patient is not depressed; a score of 5–10 indicates the presence of mild depression; and 11+ indicates major depression. Elderly patients with major depression are more likely to commit suicide than younger patients with depression.

POSTNATAL DEPRESSION

It is normal to get the 'baby blues' shortly after the birth of a baby, lasting for up to 10 days. However, persisting low mood should be investigated. Postnatal depression affects about 10% of women, often resulting in immense strain on or breakdown of family relationships. Around 5% of women are still depressed at 6 months and about 3% go on to develop chronic depression. Unsurprisingly, postnatal depression is more common in women who have been depressed during their pregnancy and in women with poor social support networks or bad marriages.

The Edinburgh Postnatal Depression Scale (EPDS) was published in the *British Journal of Psychiatry* in 1987 (volume **150**) by J.L. Cox, J.M. Holden and R. Sagovsky. It is a well-validated screening tool used to detect postnatal depression and is usually used at the 6- to 8-week postnatal check. It consists of ten questions, each with four possible responses; the woman should underline the response which most closely matches her feelings in the past 7 days (ie not just on the day of the test). No one else should complete the questionnaire on behalf of the woman unless language is an issue. The questionnaire should be used tactfully, and with a full explanation of why it is useful; otherwise, many women may feel that it is unacceptably intrusive and lose confidence in their doctor.

1   I have been able to laugh and see the funny side of things

- As much as I always could

- Not quite so much now

- Definitely not so much now

- Not at all

2   I have looked forward with enjoyment to things

- As much as I always did

- Rather less than I did

- Definitely less than I did

- Hardly at all

3 I have blamed myself unnecessarily when things went wrong

- Yes, most of the time
- Yes, some of the time
- Not very often
- No, never

4 I have been anxious or worried for no good reason

- No, not at all
- Hardly ever
- Yes, sometimes
- Yes, very often

5 I have felt scared or panicky for no very good reason

- Yes, quite a lot
- Yes, sometimes
- No, not much
- No, not at all

6 Things have been getting on top of me

- Yes, most of the time I haven't been able to cope at all
- Yes, sometimes I haven't been coping as well as usual
- No, most of the time I have coped quite well
- No, I have been coping as well as ever

7 I have been so unhappy that I have had difficulty in sleeping

- Yes, most of the time
- Yes, sometimes
- Not very often
- No, not at all

8 I have felt sad or miserable

- Yes, most of the time
- Yes, quite often
- Not very often
- No, not at all

9 I have been so unhappy that I have been crying

- Yes, most of the time
- Yes, quite often
- Only occasionally
- No, never

10 The thought of harming myself has occurred to me

- Yes, quite often
- Sometimes
- Hardly ever
- Never

The answers are all marked on a scale of 0–3, with 3 marks being given to the most severe depressive symptoms. The total score is calculated by adding up all the individual scores and is out of a maximum of 30.

Treatment with an SSRI is probably about as effective as cognitive behavioural therapy.

- Atypical drugs are known to cause weight gain and olanzapine and risperidone have been shown to increase the risk of cerebrovascular accident (CVA; see Chapter 2, Dementia). Olanzapine can lead to worsening of glycaemic control and may increase the risk of developing type 2 diabetes.

Medication should be continued for at least 1 year after the first episode of psychosis, providing that treatment has been instigated within 1 month of the onset of symptoms. If the psychosis is recurrent or more than 1 month has elapsed since diagnosis, treatment should be continued for at least 2 years. If the medication is going to be withdrawn, it should be done slowly, over at least 6–8 weeks.

	Causes sedation?	EPSEs	Weight gain	Available as im injection?	Initial dose
Amisulpride	(+)	+	+	No	200 mg bd (or 50 mg bd if mainly negative sx)
Olanzapine	++	+	+++	Not licensed	10 mg od
Quetiapine	++	–	+	No	25 mg bd day 1 50 mg bd day 2 100 mg bd day 3 150 mg bd day 4
Risperidone	+	+ (++ at high doses)	+	Yes	2 mg od day 1 4 mg od day 2
Zotepine	++	–	++	No	25 mg tds, increasing to 50 mg tds on day 4
Haloperidol	++	+++		Yes	1–2 mg bd
Chlorpromazine	+++	++		Yes	50–100 mg bd
Sulpiride	+	+		No	200 mg bd

Table 14.6: Drug treatments in schizophrenia

PHYSICAL ILLNESS IN PATIENTS WITH SCHIZOPHRENIA

A high percentage of patients with schizophrenia smoke cigarettes, drink excessive alcohol and have a poor diet. In addition to this, high-risk sexual behaviour is more common amongst schizophrenics than it is in the general population. Unsurprisingly therefore, these patients are more at risk of physical illness, including cardiovascular disease, diabetes mellitus, hyperlipidaemia, respiratory disease, hepatitis C, HIV and osteoporosis.

COMPULSORY ADMISSION UNDER THE MENTAL HEALTH ACT

Compulsory admission for assessment and/or treatment can only be considered when:

- there is a mental disorder of a nature or degree that warrants detention in hospital for assessment or treatment **and**

- it is in the interests of the health and safety of the patient **or**

- it is necessary in order to protect others.

Determining whether there is a 'mental disorder' relies on clinical judgement. If a patient is very distressed or ill, they can be sectioned even if they are not considered to be at immediate risk of harming themselves or others. Compulsory admission is always a last resort, to be used only when all other options have been exhausted.

SECTION 4

This is only used in genuine emergencies, ie when there is an immediate and significant risk of harm to the patient or to others, when there is a significant risk to the property or when the patient needs to be physically restrained. If this occurs, the GP should contact the duty approved social worker (ASW) to discuss the case and arrange admission. It may be necessary to call out the police, and an ambulance will almost certainly be required.

A section 4 requires an application by the patient's nearest relative or an ASW, using statutory forms 5 or 6 respectively. The doctor (usually the GP) will need to examine the patient and fill out statutory form 7 (the medical recommendation form), which can be obtained from the ASW or directly from the Department of Social Security (DSS). If there is no ASW involved, the GP will need copies of both application form 5 and recommendation form 7. A bed will need to be arranged at a local psychiatric unit and admission must take place within 24 hours of the examination. Form 14 is also necessary for any section: this details the medical recommendations and is a formal record of admission.

If the patient is about to injure himself, herself or others, it is defensible to give emergency treatment under common law. This would usually be with a sedative such as lorazepam 1–4 mg orally or as an im injection. If treatment is to be given forcibly, the police would need to be involved in order to restrain the patient.

A section 4 lasts for up to 72 hours.

SECTION 2

Section 2 is used when the diagnosis is unclear and there is no treatment plan in place. It allows for the compulsory detention of the patient for an assessment period of up to 28 days. An approved psychiatrist and ASW or relative are needed, in addition to the patient's usual doctor (or failing this, another section 12(2) approved doctor). The statutory forms required are forms 1 or 2 (application forms to be filled in by the patient's nearest relative or by the ASW respectively) and forms 3 (a joint medical recommendation form) or 4 (for separate medical recommendations, when the psychiatrist and GP are unable to examine the patient at the same time). If there is no ASW available, the GP will need to bring copies of forms 1 and 4 with them.

Ideally, the psychiatrist and GP will examine the patient at the same time, but, failing this, the examinations are legally allowed to be up to 5 days apart.

SECTION 3

Section 3 is a treatment order and can last for up to 6 months. It specifies the category of mental disorder and is usually reserved for patients who are already known to the psychiatric services. It can only be used for patients with treatable conditions. The patient is allowed to make an appeal to the Mental Health Review Tribunal within 6 months of admission and then subsequently once each time the section is extended.

SECTION 136

This allows a police officer to remove a mentally disordered patient from a public place to a place of safety (such as a hospital or police station).

SECTION 135

This is used when an ASW wishes to remove a patient from their home to a place of safety, but is unable to gain access: the ASW must apply for a magistrate's warrant authorising them to enter the patient's home. The ASW will usually be accompanied by a police officer and the patient's GP.

MENTAL HEALTH AND THE NEW GMS CONTRACT

In order to achieve maximum quality points, the following standards must be met:

- The practice must be able to produce a register of patients with severe, long-term mental health problems who require and have agreed to regular follow-up.

- 90% of these patients must have had a comprehensive review in the past 15 months, including a check on their physical health, a medication review and a review of secondary care arrangements.

- 90% of patients on lithium must have had their lithium levels checked in the past 6 months and a creatinine level and thyroid functions done in the past 15 months; 70% of patients on lithium must have had lithium levels in the therapeutic range within the past 6 months.

COGNITIVE BEHAVIOURAL THERAPY (CBT)

This section is only intended to be a very basic introduction to an extremely complicated area. There are many different types of psychological therapies available, but CBT is probably the most well-researched and is considered to be reasonably cost-effective. The basic premise behind CBT is that events that occur in life lead to thoughts, which in turn result in feelings and behaviour. Negative thoughts can result in destructive behaviour. People think negatively as a direct result of their life experiences and core beliefs about themselves; these core beliefs are shaped in early childhood. By being aware of negative thoughts, 'separating' them from the event and the mood, and objectively analysing them, outcomes for the patient can be improved.

Common examples of negative thought processes include:

- 'Jumping to conclusions', where the patient is convinced without evidence that somebody thinks badly of them, or believes from the outset that things will not work out for them.

- 'Helplessness', when the patient believes that they do not have the power to change their situation and are effectively at the mercy of external influences.

- Disregarding positive events: ignoring compliments and achievements and focusing only on the negative.

- 'All or nothing' thinking: thinking that if something isn't entirely perfect or fully completed, that they have failed entirely.

- Generalisation: feeling that one mistake, failure or particular shortcoming means that success in other areas is not possible.

- Overreacting in an emotional way to fairly trivial events, and perhaps 'blowing them up out of all proportion'.

- Accepting blame for things which may not be their fault.

- Having overexacting expectations of the way things 'should' work, or the way in which people 'should' behave, which will always lead to disappointment and resentment.

People can fall into a pattern of always thinking in a negative way, which may then result in depression or anger. This can be because of generally low self-esteem (a core belief), caused for example by childhood events such as abuse or neglect or being raised by over-critical parents. It can sometimes take prolonged and intensive therapy to overcome these underlying beliefs, which the patient may not be consciously aware of at all.

It is often helpful to encourage depressed patients to keep a 'thought diary' in which they record the adverse event, how they felt because of it and their initial, 'automatic' thoughts, memories or impressions. Just being aware of these thoughts can raise the patient's self awareness.

For example:

Situation/event	Feelings	'Automatic' thoughts or images
Friday evening. I have suggested that two of my colleagues come out for a drink with me after work. Neither of them can make it.	Embarrassed Worthless Angry	They don't want to spend time with me They don't like me I didn't have many friends at school No one likes me even now I am not a likeable person

In this case, the patient has overreacted to what most people would think of as a minor incident, possibly because of low self-esteem as a result of being unpopular at school. This has led them to reach the conclusion that they are unlovable and that life is 'unfair'. These thoughts, rather than the situation per se, are what make them feel unhappy and resentful. The patient may become wary of feeling this way again, and so become more socially isolated (a negative behaviour), which in turn exacerbates any underlying depression.

When the patient has become accustomed to recording their thoughts in this way after any adverse event, they should be asked to weigh up the evidence for and against their thoughts and to reassess their interpretation of the situation. For example, in the above scenario, evidence against the patient's thoughts might be found by remembering previous social contact with their colleagues or by taking into consideration the short notice of their invitation. Reflecting on this may lead to an alteration in some of their thoughts, for example they may now come to the conclusion that their colleagues have always been friendly in the past, and that there is no evidence to support their initial thoughts. This realisation might help to lift their mood.

For example:

Evidence that supports the thought	Evidence that does not support the thought	New, 'balanced' thoughts	Mood
I find it difficult to make friends	My colleagues have always been friendly in the past, and seem to like me	It is possible that it wasn't because my colleagues don't like me that they said no; perhaps they just had other plans	More optimistic
I am shy	One has a family and may have other commitments		
I had a difficult time at school			

Behavioural techniques can also help with depression, for example asking the patient to plan at least one enjoyable event for each day, perhaps something as simple as taking a walk. People who avoid social contact altogether should make sure that they engage in some type of interaction daily, even if it is simply something like asking a stranger for the time.

CBT can help with anxiety as well. Most people experience a certain level of anxiety in stressful situations. Anxiety causes release of adrenaline, which produces physical symptoms such as tachycardia, sweating, etc, the so-called 'flight or fight' response. Often, panic and fear are caused by a subconscious misinterpretation of these physical symptoms, which culminates in the patient thinking that something catastrophic is going to happen to them, for example that they are going to die, faint, lose control, go mad or do something very embarrassing. It is this 'catastrophising' that leads to the symptoms of uncontrollable anxiety experienced in a panic attack.

For example:

Situation/event	Feelings	'Automatic thoughts'
Tuesday morning. I have to give a presentation to my team at work. There will be ten of us, including my boss	Panic	I am bad at speaking in public
	Intense anxiety	Everyone will think I am stupid I can feel my heart racing I am sweating My chest feels tight I am going to vomit in front of all my colleagues

On a practical note, understanding (and believing) that the symptoms experienced do not equate with any physical danger and will not lead to catastrophe can help with feelings of anxiety; patients should think back to all the times in the past when they have been anxious and convinced that they were going to be physically unwell. Even when they were experiencing intense symptoms of anxiety, they will realise that they have remained physically well and that they have never 'lost control'. Some people are reassured by an explanation of the physiological changes that occur when they are anxious. Beta-blockers can sometimes be used to help mask the symptoms.

The underlying fear that leads to the physical symptoms can also be dealt with and behavioural strategies may be useful. In this case, it might help to present the work to just one colleague at a time on several occasions, so that when it comes to presenting in front of more than one person, the patient knows that 'they can do it'; then, when they are analysing the evidence for and against their fear of failure (as in the first example), they can take into account these past successes.

OTHER STRATEGIES TO HELP DEAL WITH ANXIETY

- **'Controlled breathing'**: the patient should be told to breathe in and out through their nose slowly, and from their diaphragm rather than the chest ('nose, low and slow'). Suggesting a slightly longer exhalation rate may help – eg breathe in to a count of four, exhale to a count of five or six, then pause for a count of two before starting the cycle again. This needs to be repeated several times (possibly for a few minutes) before the patient will notice any improvement in their levels of anxiety.

- **Relaxation techniques**: yoga and meditation can be very helpful.

- **Exercise**: regular exercise may be a useful outlet for people with chronic anxiety.

- **Imagery**: visualising a pleasant, relaxing scene at times of stress.

- **Distraction techniques**: trying to focus 'out' rather than 'in' when in a stressful situation, eg closely observing the people or objects in their immediate environment.

- **Facing fears**: patients with specific anxieties usually avoid coming into contact with the source of their anxiety, eg flying, making speeches. By trying to face these fears instead of simply avoiding them, anxiety can be definitively dealt with. Usually, patients should be encouraged to use a graduated approach. For example, someone who is frightened of using the underground should travel one or two stops at a time, and slowly build up journey times. They can use the techniques discussed here to help them.

An excellent self-help book is *Mind over Mood* by Dennis Greenberger and Christine Padesky, published by Guilford Press (1995).

A useful website is the Australian 'mood gym' site (www.moodgym.anu.edu.au).

CHAPTER 15
RESPIRATORY MEDICINE

CHAPTER 15
RESPIRATORY MEDICINE

ASTHMA

The latest British Thoracic Society guidelines came out in 2003 and were updated in 2004. Some points of note are listed below.

- The guidelines recommend that inhaled steroids (at a dose of 400 micrograms/day of beclomethasone in adults or 200 micrograms/day in children) should be considered if a patient has had an exacerbation of their asthma in the past 2 years **or** if they are symptomatic, needing a beta-agonist at least three times a week **or** if they are symptomatic at least one night per week. Exercise-induced asthma is often (but not always) a sign of poor control.

- Beclomethasone is equivalent to budesonide in terms of dosage, and a 1:1 ratio should be assumed when changing from one to the other. There is limited evidence that using the budesonide Turbohaler® results in greater lung deposition compared with other devices. Fluticasone provides equivalent clinical activity to beclomethasone and budesonide at half the dosage: for example, 400 micrograms/day of beclomethasone is equivalent to 200 micrograms fluticasone.

- There is no difference in efficacy between giving inhaled steroids and long-acting beta$_2$-agonists in combination or as separate inhalers.

- Inhaled steroids are often used in inappropriately high dosages; the patient should always be maintained on the lowest effective dose. In general, for patients who are stable, the dose of inhaled steroid should be reduced by 25–50% every 3 months.

- Patients who are considered to require inhaled steroids should initially be started off on a moderate dose, eg 400 micrograms beclomethasone.

- Inhaled steroids are thought to be safe in doses of <800 micrograms beclomethasone per day for adults and <400 micrograms beclomethasone per day for children. Adults who regularly take higher doses may be at increased risk of osteoporosis and children may be at risk of short-term growth suppression or adrenal insufficiency.

- In terms of monitoring patients with asthma, there is increasing evidence (*Journal of General Internal Medicine* 2004; **19**: 237–42) that asking about quality of life indicators is better than measuring peak flow in terms of predicting an exacerbation. Questions recommended by the Royal College of Physicians are:

  - Have you had your usual asthma symptoms during the day?

  - Have you had any difficulty in sleeping because of your asthma?

  - Has your asthma interfered with your usual activities?

- The British Thoracic Society no longer recommends that the patient should double their dose of inhaled steroid during an asthma exacerbation, due to lack of evidence of efficacy (*Thorax* 2004; **59**: 550–6; *Lancet* 2004; **363**: 271–5). However, in practice, many patients feel that there is benefit in doing this. Interestingly, asthma self-management plans that include doubling the dose of inhaled steroid when the patient deteriorates have been shown to improve asthma control. Some experts recommend that the patient should actually treble or quadruple their inhaled steroid for up to 2 weeks during an exacerbation.

- Asthmatics are at increased risk of developing chronic obstructive pulmonary disease (COPD) in later life.

THE GMS CONTRACT AND ASTHMA

To achieve maximum quality points, the following standards need to be met:

- The practice must have an up-to-date register of asthmatic patients (excluding those who have not been prescribed asthma-related drugs in the past year).

- 70% of adults and children older than 8 years should have had their diagnosis confirmed by serial peak flows or spirometry.

- 70% of patients older than 14 years need to have an up-to-date record of their smoking status within the previous 15 months (the exception being adults who have never smoked, who only need to have their status recorded once).

- 70% of asthmatics who smoke should have been offered smoking cessation advice within the past 15 months.

- 70% of asthmatics should have had an annual review within the past 15 months.

- 70% of asthmatics older than 16 years should have an annual influenza vaccination.

TYPES OF INHALER

There are two types of asthma inhalers: aerosol inhalers and dry powder inhalers.

Aerosol inhalers include **autohalers**, which are breath-actuated (eg Salamol Easi-Breathe®, Beclazone Easi-Breathe®, Qvar Autohaler®) and the traditional **metered-dose inhalers**. Autohalers can be prescribed for adults and children over the age of 5 years who have an inspiratory flow of at least 30 litres per minute. They tend to be associated with high oropharyngeal deposition. Patients who are prescribed autohalers should be given the following instructions:

1 Remove the cap from the mouthpiece.

2 Lift the grey lever at the top of the autohaler and shake the inhaler well, holding it upright.

3 Exhale fully, and then place the inhaler in your mouth, creating a tight seal.

4 Breathe in though your mouth, slowly and deeply, for about 5 seconds. The autohaler automatically releases a dose of the medication.

5 Hold your breath for 10 seconds.

6 Breathe out slowly through your nose and return the grey lever to its original position.

The mouthpiece needs to be cleaned at least once per week, usually with a dry tissue (check manufacturer's instructions).

Metered-dose inhalers are not usually prescribed to children under the age of 11 years. They are less expensive than other devices and can be used with a spacer. A greater degree of coordination is required, in that the patient needs to press down on the metal canister just after they start to breathe in. They then continue to breathe in and hold their breath for 10 seconds at maximal inspiration. The mouthpiece needs to be removed from the metal canister and cleaned once a week with warm running water. It should be allowed to air-dry.

DRY POWDER INHALERS

These can be used in adults and in most children above the age of 5 years.

Pros

- No coordination required

- Pleasant/no taste

- Shape/colour may appeal to teenagers (although shape of turbohaler may not be ideal for teenage girls!)

- The patient can tell when it is empty.

Cons

- More expensive than metered-dose inhalers

- Still require a reasonable amount of inspiratory effort to trigger the device (at least 30 litres/minute for an accuhaler and 60 litres/minute for a turbohaler)

- Cannot be used with a spacer, so not good for acute attacks, when the patient does not have sufficient respiratory reserve left to trigger the device.

Dry powder devices include:

- **Turbohalers** (eg budesonide, Symbicort®, Oxis®, terbutaline). The patient needs to unscrew the turbohaler and lift off its cap. They then twist the coloured base of the device to the right, and then the left, until it clicks. They need to exhale fully (away from the device), then put the mouthpiece into their mouth (ensuring a good seal) and breathe in through their mouth as forcefully as they can manage, for about 5 seconds. Finally, they should remove the turbohaler from their mouth before breathing out. The turbohaler contains 200 doses of medication and the indicator on its side appears red when it is empty.

- **Accuhalers** (eg fluticasone, salmeterol, Seretide®). These are circular devices containing 60 doses of medication; there is a counter that indicates how many doses are left. The accuhaler needs to be held in the base of one hand, with the thumb of the other hand resting in the thumb grip. The inhaler is opened by pushing the thumb grip round, until it clicks. The patient should exhale, and then put the mouthpiece firmly in their mouth, ensuring a good seal, and breathe in steadily for about 5 seconds. They should then hold their breath for 10 seconds before exhaling and closing the accuhaler.

Dry powder devices should always be held upright when loading the medication, so that the powder does not fall out. They should be kept away from moisture and the patient should not blow into them. There is always a way of telling how much medication is left and the patient should be instructed to check this regularly.

SPACER DEVICES

Spacers are recommended for use in children up to the age of 5 years. Children under the age of 2 years will need a face mask as well as a spacer. They are also recommended for patients with severe COPD and in patients who are on high doses of inhaled steroids:

- >400 micrograms beclomethasone (or 200 micrograms fluticasone) per day in children younger than 5 years old

- >800 micrograms (or 500 micrograms fluticasone) per day in adults or children older than 5 years old.

USING A SPACER - PRACTICAL POINTS

- The dose should be inhaled within 10 seconds of activating the metered-dose inhaler (MDI), as settling of the drug reduces deposition.

- The spacer should be washed with washing-up liquid about once every 2 weeks, and allowed to drip-dry.

- Single actuations (repeated as necessary) should be used rather than multiple actuations, and the canister should be shaken between each actuation.

- After each actuation, the patient should breathe in and out normally for about four to five breaths.

- Face masks should be placed firmly over the mouth and nose, to create a good seal.

- Some spacers need to be tilted upwards by about 10° when used in babies, in order to open the valve; older children should have enough inspiratory effort to manage this anyway.

- Different spacer devices are compatible with different inhalers.

- Manufacturers recommend that the Volumatic® and Nebuhaler® are replaced every 6 months (although in practice spacers usually last longer than this) and AeroChambers® every year.

- Spacers with large chambers, eg the Volumatic®, work better than smaller spacers.

Spacer device	Compatible inhalers
Volumatic®	Salbutamol, salmeterol, fluticasone, beclomethasone, Seretide®
AeroChamber®	Salbutamol, terbutaline, salmeterol, fluticasone, beclomethasone, budesonide, Seretide®, Symbicort®, Atrovent®
Able Spacer®	Salbutamol, terbutaline, salmeterol, fluticasone, beclomethasone, budesonide, Seretide®, Symbicort®, Atrovent®
Nebuhaler®	Terbutaline, budesonide, Symbicort®, Atrovent®

Table 15.1: Spacer devices and their compatible inhalers

* Beclomethasone propionate (BDP) or equivalent
† Higher nominal doses may be required if drug delivery is difficult

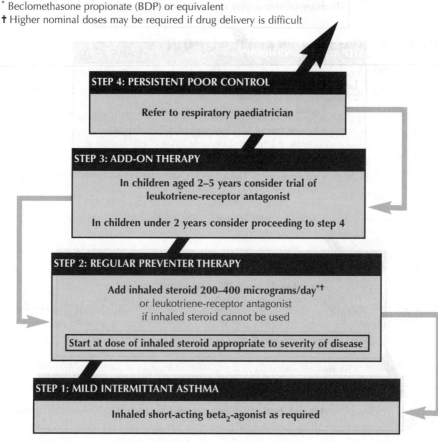

Figure 15.1. Management of asthma in children under 5 years old (with copyright permission: *British Guideline on the management of Asthma*, Revised Edition, British Thoracic Society, 2004, p.28)

British Thoracic Society guidelines on the management of asthma, are summarised in Figures 15.1, 15.2 and 15.3.

* BDP or equivalent

STEP 5: CONTINUOUS OR FREQUENT USE OF ORAL STEROIDS

Use daily steroid tablet in lowest dose providing adequate control
Maintain high-dose inhaled steroid at 800 micrograms/day*
Refer to respiratory paediatrician

STEP 4: PERSISTENT POOR CONTROL

Increase inhaled steroid up to 800 micrograms/day*

STEP 3: ADD-ON THERAPY

1 **Add inhaled long-acting beta$_2$ -agonist (LABA)**
2 **Assess control of asthma:**
  - **good response** to LABA – continue LABA

  - **benefit from LABA but control still inadequate** – continue LABA and increase inhaled steroid dose to 400 micrograms/day* (if not already on this dose)

  - **no response to LABA** – stop LABA and increase inhaled steroid to 400 micrograms/day.* If control still inadequate, institute trial of other therapies, eg leukotriene-receptor antagonist or SR theophylline

STEP 2: REGULAR PREVENTER THERAPY

Add inhaled steroid 200–400 micrograms/day*
(other preventer drug if inhaled steroid cannot be used)
200 micrograms is an appropriate starting dose for many patients

Start at dose of inhaled steroid appropriate to severity of disease

STEP 1: MILD INTERMITTENT ASTHMA

Inhaled short-acting beta$_2$-agonist as required

Figure 15.2 Management of asthma in children aged 5–12 years (with copyright permission: *British Guideline on the management of Asthma*, Revised Edition, British Thoracic Society, 2004, p.27)

STEP 5: CONTINUOUS OR FREQUENT US OF ORAL STEROIDS

Use daily steroid tablet in lowest dose providing adequate control
Maintain high-dose inhaled steroid at 2000 micrograms/day*
Consider other treatments to minimise the use of steroid tablets
Refer patient for specialist care

STEP 4: PERSISTANT POOR CONTROL

Consider trials of:
• Increasing inhaled steroid up to 2000 micrograms/day*

• Addition of a fourth drug – eg leukotriene receptor antagonist, SR theophylline, beta$_2$-agonist tablet

STEP 3: ADD-ON THERAPY

1 Add inhaled long-acting beta$_2$-agonist (LABA)
2 Assess control of asthma:
• good response to LABA – continue LABA

• benefit from LABA but control still inadequate – continue LABA and increase inhaled steroid dose to 800 micrograms/day* (if not already on this dose)

• no response to LABA – stop LABA and increase inhaled steroid to 800 micrograms/day.* If control still inadequate, institute trial of other therapies, eg leukotriene-receptor antagonist or SR theophylline

STEP 2: REGULAR PREVENTER THERAPY

Add inhaled steroid 200–800micrograms/day*

400 micrograms is an appropriate starting dose for many patients

Start at dose of inhaled steroid appropriate to severity of disease

STEP 1: MILD INTERMITTENT ASTHMA

Inhaled short-acting beta$_2$-agonist as required

* BDP or equivalent

Figure 15.3 Management of asthma in adults (with copyright permission: *British Guideline on the management of Asthma*, Revised Edition, British Thoracic Society, 2004, p.26)

CHRONIC OBSTRUCTIVE PULMONARY DISEASE (COPD)

COPD should be considered in any smoker over 35 who presents with a cough or shortness of breath. It is, however, less likely if a patient who gave up smoking many years ago and who was previously asymptomatic reports new-onset dyspnoea. Spirometry provides a definitive diagnosis although according to new NICE guidance, anybody with a persistant, unexplained cough should also be referred for a chest X-ray.

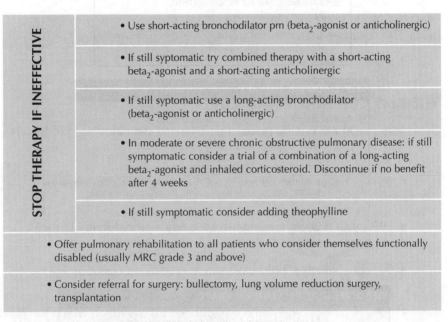

STOP THERAPY IF INEFFECTIVE

- Use short-acting bronchodilator prn (beta$_2$-agonist or anticholinergic)

- If still syptomatic try combined therapy with a short-acting beta$_2$-agonist and a short-acting anticholinergic

- If still syptomatic use a long-acting bronchodilator (beta$_2$-agonist or anticholinergic)

- In moderate or severe chronic obstructive pulmonary disease: if still symptomatic consider a trial of a combination of a long-acting beta$_2$-agonist and inhaled corticosteroid. Discontinue if no benefit after 4 weeks

- If still symptomatic consider adding theophylline

- Offer pulmonary rehabilitation to all patients who consider themselves functionally disabled (usually MRC grade 3 and above)

- Consider referral for surgery: bullectomy, lung volume reduction surgery, transplantation

Figure 15.4 Management of COPD (NICE 2004)

The 2004 NICE guidelines summarise the management of COPD (Figure 15.4). Patients with moderate or severe COPD (ie with a forced expiratory volume in 1 second (FEV$_1$) <50% of the predicted normal) no longer need formal assessment with spirometry to see whether they will benefit from long-term inhaled steroids; it is sufficient for the clinician to assess this on the basis of symptoms. Patients with an FEV$_1$ of <50% of the predicted normal measure who have had more than two exacerbations in the past year and those whose symptoms are not controlled with a combination of short- and long-acting bronchodilators can be given a 4-week trial of inhaled steroids; if they feel better on this, it can be continued.

Lifestyle changes, in particular weight loss and smoking cessation, are vital. Depression is common in COPD patients and should not be overlooked.

HOME OXYGEN

By the end of 2005, prescription of home oxygen for patients with COPD is likely to take place in a secondary care setting. Patients with long-standing hypoxaemia and an arterial oxygen tension (PaO_2) of less than 7.3 kPa (or <8 kPa in the presence of pulmonary hypertension, peripheral oedema or nocturnal hypoxaemia) will probably derive most benefit from at least 15 hours of oxygen per day, delivered via a concentrator. However, there is also a role for ambulatory oxygen treatment in selected patients, for example those who are shown to be able to walk significantly further with the help of oxygen. Concentrators are more cost-effective than cylinders if oxygen is being used for more than 8 hours per day.

Patients should be referred to secondary care for initiation of oxygen therapy.

THE GMS CONTRACT AND COPD

To achieve maximum quality points, the following standards need to be met:

- The practice must have a register of COPD patients.
- 90% of patients should have had their diagnosis confirmed by spirometry.
- 90% of COPD patients should have had a record made of their smoking status within the past 15 months.
- 90% of smokers should have received smoking cessation advice within the past 15 months.
- 70% of patients should have had their FEV_1 recorded within the past 27 months.
- 90% of patients should have had their inhaler technique checked in the past 2 years.
- 85% of COPD patients should receive an influenza immunisation.

CHAPTER 16
RHEUMATOLOGY

CHAPTER 16
RHEUMATOLOGY

RHEUMATOID ARTHRITIS

DIAGNOSTIC CRITERIA

The American College of Rheumatology (ACR) criteria for the classification of rheumatoid arthritis (RA) are widely accepted. However, they are mainly used in research and are less useful in routine clinical practice (for example, patients with early disease may be missed). Diagnosis of RA requires four out of the following seven criteria:

- Morning stiffness of at least 1 hour for >6 weeks
- Arthritis with swelling of three or more joint areas for >6 weeks
- Arthritis with swelling of hand (metacarpophalangeal (MCP) or proximal interphalangeal (PIP) joints) or wrist joints for >6 weeks
- Symmetrical arthritis of at least one part of the body (eg elbows, wrists, knees) for >6 weeks
- Subcutaneous nodules
- Serum rheumatoid factor-positive (occurs in 70–80% of cases, but is also positive in other diseases, such as systemic lupus erythematosus (SLE) and polymyositis)
- Typical radiographic features of hand or wrist with erosions or peri-articular osteopenia (although X-rays are often normal in early disease).

Rheumatoid arthritis most often presents in the fifth decade and is more common in women. The most usual presentation is of a symmetrical arthritis affecting the PIP joints of both hands, worse in the morning and lasting for at least 6 weeks. Prompt referral is important, as early introduction of disease-modifying drugs (eg methotrexate, sulfasalazine, azathioprine and hydroxychloroquine) may be able to limit irreversible joint damage.

INTERPRETING RHEUMATOID FACTOR RESULTS

These results refer to the factor by which serum has to be diluted before the antibodies can no longer be detected, ie 1:40 means that the serum has to be diluted by a factor of 40 before detection can no longer take place, while a result of 1:160 means that the serum has to be diluted 160 times before the antibodies disappear. Therefore, the higher the second number, the more strongly positive the result is, and the worse the prognosis:

- A value of <1:40 is negative.

- A value of between 1:40 and 1:80 is borderline.

- A significantly raised rheumatoid factor is one of above 1:160.

- The same applies when interpreting other autoantibody results, eg antinuclear antibody (ANA).

TREATMENT AND PROGNOSIS

More than 50% of patients will not become disabled and will remain independent. Some people recover completely after one or two minor flare-ups and some continue to experience intermittent flare-ups but with little or no residual disability. A minority experience progressive symptoms that result in permanent pain and disability. Newly diagnosed patients should normally be referred to a rheumatologist to decide whether to initiate disease-modifying antirheumatic drugs (DMARDs). Treatment will usually consist of the following:

- **NSAIDS**: different NSAIDs work for different patients, so it is worth trying a selection. About a third of patients derive considerable benefit from NSAIDs, a third experience a degree of improvement and a third do not respond. A long-acting NSAID such as modified-release diclofenac may be helpful at night. If there has been no response to an NSAID within 3 weeks, it is worth switching to a different one.

- **Steroids**: long-term steroids are rarely indicated and their most common use is in the short term, for treatment of acute exacerbations.

- **Disease-modifying antirheumatic drugs (DMARDs)**: these drugs reduce joint inflammation and are often introduced early on in the course of treatment. They can take up to 6 months to take full effect (although a beneficial effect is usually observed after 1–3 months) and may be used for several years. There are many different drugs to choose from, including methotrexate, sulfasalazine, azathioprine and leflunomide. Blood monitoring is usually necessary (see also Chapter 6, Gastroenterology).

Methotrexate	Full blood count (FBC) weekly for the first 6 weeks, then monthly
	Liver function tests (LFTs) 3-monthly
	FBC 1 week after any change in dosage

Table 16.1: Testing required while on methotrexate

POLYMYALGIA RHEUMATICA (PMR)

PMR lasts on average for 2–3 years. The mean age of onset is 70 years, and disease before the age of 50 is very rare. It is more common in female Caucasians.

DIAGNOSIS

- Bilateral shoulder and pelvic girdle pain
- Symptoms lasting >2 months
- Initial erythrocyte sedimentation rate (ESR) of >30 mm/hour
- Morning stiffness lasting >1 hour
- No signs of muscular disease, RA, inflammatory arthritis or malignant disease.

Patients often complain of fatigue, weight loss and anorexia. Shoulder and pelvic girdle pain are usually worse first thing in the morning.

TREATMENT

- Start with 15 mg prednisolone and continue at this dose for 4 weeks.
- Reduce to 10 mg over another 4 weeks.
- Reduce by 1 mg every 6 weeks, and then stop altogether; if the patient relapses or the ESR starts to climb again, the steroid dose may have to be increased until the symptoms settle.

Treating PMR with steroids usually results in improvement within a few days (usually 2–4 days) rather than weeks. ESR and C-reactive protein (CRP) normalise within 1–2 weeks; if this is not the case, the diagnosis should be reconsidered. Note that the shoulders may remain stiff for months. It remains debatable whether it is better to use symptomatic improvement or declining ESR as a measure of the success of treatment. ESR is sometimes low even in active disease and therefore many experts advocate that treatment should be guided mainly by symptoms. The median duration of time for which steroids are needed is 2 years, although treatment is sometimes much more protracted.

Patients may require a small dose of NSAIDs after the steroids are stopped, to help with muscle pain. For patients who relapse after a successful course of treatment, NSAIDs alone are sometimes sufficient. If not, often lower doses of steroids will suffice (eg 5 mg).

People who initially respond to treatment but then get worse may have another condition, such as rheumatoid arthritis.

STEROIDS AND OSTEOPOROSIS

Steroids can have various side-effects, which should be monitored, such as, osteoporosis and gastritis. Anyone who is on oral steroids (at any dose) for more than 3 months needs to have their bone density assessed with a DEXA scan except:

- Those over 65 years old

- Those who have had a previous fragility fracture (defined as occurring with minimal trauma, after the age of 40 years).

These patients should automatically be started on preventative treatment with a bisphosphonate if they are given >3 months' treatment with an oral steroid. Note that this advice has changed: previously, prophylaxis was only recommended if the dose of steroid was >7.5 mg. The Royal College of Physicians of London states that oral steroids significantly increase the risk of spine and hip fractures, whatever the dose prescribed.

GOUT

Gout has a prevalence of about 1% in the UK and is most common in Caucasian men over the age of 45 (it is very rare in Black Africans). The big toe is the most common site to be affected, but other joints that may be involved include the knee, wrist and finger. Gout is more likely to occur in patients with raised serum uric acid levels (>0.42 mmol/l), but most patients with hyperuricaemia do not have gout and therefore do not need to be treated. Uric acid levels may return to normal during an acute attack.

Acute attacks of gout usually resolve within 1 or 2 weeks. Treatment is with either NSAIDs or colchicine in patients who cannot tolerate NSAIDs. Colchicine commonly produces gastrointestinal side-effects when given at licensed doses (1 mg followed by 500 micrograms every 2–3 hours until pain relief is achieved, to a maximum of 6 mg/day). Some case reports (*British Medical Journal* 2003; **327**: 1275) have suggested that smaller doses of 500 micrograms tds are just as effective, but produce fewer side-effects.

PROPHYLAXIS

Losing weight and reducing alcohol and red meat consumption tend to result in a lowering of serum uric acid concentrations, and should therefore be encouraged. Patients who have two or more attacks per year may wish to consider prophylactic treatment, particularly if they find it difficult to take NSAIDs or colchicine. Allopurinol is a xanthine oxidase inhibitor, and is the most commonly used prophylactic drug. It should usually be started at a low dose (eg 100 mg od, taken with food) and then gradually increased until the serum uric acid concentration falls into the normal range. Allopurinol should never be initiated during an acute attack of gout (it may prolong the attack). Cover with an NSAID or colchicine is necessary for at least the first 3 months of treatment. If the patient gets an acute attack while on allopurinol, the drug should be continued at the same dose, and concomitant treatment with an NSAID or colchicine should be started.

OSTEOPOROSIS

Osteoporosis is a huge public health problem: 1 in 3 women and 1 in 12 men over the age of 50 will sustain an osteoporotic fracture in their lifetime. Fifty per cent of people lose the ability to live independently following a hip fracture, and there is a 20% increase in mortality.

The Royal College of Physicians recommends DEXA scanning in the following circumstances:

- History of fragility fractures

- Kyphosis and loss of height due to vertebral crush fracture, as confirmed by radiography (people with a history of two or more vertebral fractures are automatically considered to be at high risk and should be started on prophylaxis without waiting for a DEXA scan)

- Radiographic evidence of osteopenia or vertebral deformity

- Oral steroids at any dose for >3 months (unless >65 or previous fragility fracture – then start prophylaxis regardless)

- Premature menopause (<45)

- History of amenorrhoea for >1 year

- Primary hypogonadism

- Chronic disease associated with osteoporosis, eg rheumatoid arthritis, hyperthyroidism, Crohn's disease, coeliac disease, alcoholism, anorexia nervosa

- Maternal family history of hip fracture

- Body mass index (BMI) <19 kg/m^2.

WHO SHOULD HAVE TREATMENT?

PRODIGY/SIGN guidelines 2003

- Patients who have a low bone mineral density (BMD) as confirmed by a DEXA scan, ie those with a T score of –2.5 or less with risk factors for osteoporosis (see above).

- Patients with two or more vertebral fractures.

- Patients >65 or with a history of fragility fractures who have been on prednisolone for >3 months.
- Consider bisphosphonate treatment for patients with osteopenia only if they have had a fragility fracture in the past (differs from NICE advice).

People with a T score of between –1 and –2.5 have osteopenia, and should be given lifestyle advice. If patients have a low-calcium diet, supplementation may be beneficial. People over the age of 65 should aim to have 400–800 units daily of vitamin D; this may not be possible through diet alone.

NICE has recently published guidance on secondary prophylaxis of osteoporotic fractures. This has already been criticised, as younger women with a history of fragility fractures may be denied access to treatment.

NICE guidance on secondary prevention of osteoporotic fractures 2005

Bisphosphonates are recommended for the following groups of patients with a history of fragility fracture:

- Women aged >75 without the need for a DEXA scan
- Women aged 65–74 if osteoporosis is confirmed by DEXA scan, (if there is a high index of clinical suspicion, treatment may be commenced once the woman has been referred for a DEXA scan and stopped later if necessary once the results of the scan are available)
- Postmenopausal women aged <65 with a T score <–3.2 or <–2.5 if there is an additional risk factor (eg history of maternal hip fracture, BMI of <19 kg/m^2, the patient is a smoker, there is a history of corticosteroid use or premature menopause, or if the patient has a disease that affects bone metabolism).

NICE does not recommend using a bisphosphonate if the T score is >–2.5, even if there is a history of fragility fractures. This is different from current guidance.

WHICH DRUG TO PRESCRIBE?

It is important to note that drugs alone are not going to be effective in patients who have a history of recurrent falls; underling causes should also be addressed (see below).

Bisphosphonates

There is most evidence for alendronate (in men and women) and risedronate (in women only). Patients who have had a history of achalasia or strictures, or those who cannot tolerate these drugs could be offered cyclical etidronate. However, unlike alendronate and risedronate, etidronate does not reduce the risk of non-vertebral fractures. Age alone should not be a reason to withhold bisphosphonates, but they are not routinely prescribed for women of child-bearing age or for pregnant women. Patients should be advised that bisphosphonates are very poorly absorbed and must be taken on an empty stomach in order to maximise their absorption.

Raloxifene

Raloxifene is an alternative to the bisphosphonates, but does not reduce the risk of non-vertebral fractures; it does, however, protect against breast cancer, although there is an increased risk of thromboembolic disease associated with its use. In their draft guidance, NICE recommends it for secondary prevention in women for whom bisphosphonates are contraindicated, for those who are physically unable to take a bisphosphonate in the recommended manner, and for women who have had an inadequate clinical response to, or who are intolerant of, bisphosphonates. A clinically inadequate response is defined as sustaining a further fracture even after 2–3 years of adequate treatment.

Hormone replacement therapy (HRT)

HRT may be considered if a woman is symptomatic from the menopause and has osteopenia, but it is not licensed to treat established osteoporosis.

Calcitonin

Calcitonin (used intranasally) is a newer medication. However, it is very expensive and has not been shown to reduce the risk of non-vertebral fractures.

Parathyroid hormone (teriparatide)

Parathyroid hormone (teriparatide) was approved in the UK for the treatment of severe osteoporosis in postmenopausal women in June 2003. The recommended dose is 20 µg administered once daily by subcutaneous injection into the thigh or abdomen. Patients taking teriparatide must receive training on the injection technique. The maximum total duration of treatment should not exceed 18 months, because of concerns about its carcinogenic potential (in rats only!). NICE recommends that it should only be used in secondary prevention of osteoporotic fractures for women >65 who have not responded to treatment with bisphosphonates (or who are intolerant to them) **and** who have a very high fracture risk (T score <–4.0; or <–3.0 if there is a history of multiple fractures **plus** one or more of the following risk factors: maternal history of hip fracture under the age of 75, BMI <19 kg/m^2, prolonged immobility or untreated premature menopause).

Calcium and vitamin D

Calcium (600–1200 mg daily) and vitamin D (400–800 units daily) supplements are often given in conjunction with bisphosphonates, particularly if the patient has a poor diet. All frail and housebound patients (eg in nursing and residential homes) should probably be considered for treatment. NICE advises that, 'unless the clinician is confident that women who receive osteoporosis treatment have an adequate calcium intake and are vitamin D replete, calcium and/or vitamin D supplementation should be provided.

Strontium ranelate

Strontium ranelate works by suppressing the action of osteoclasts and by stimulating osteoblasts. Its precise place in treatment is not well established and there have not yet been any studies comparing it with other osteoporosis medications in terms of effectiveness in reducing the risk of fractures.

SECONDARY OSTEOPOROSIS

Osteoporosis in men (particularly under the age of 65) and in premenopausal women usually has an underlying cause, such as hyperthyroidism, hypogonadism, malabsorption (coeliac disease, chronic liver disease, inflammatory bowel disease, anorexia), drugs (corticosteroids and medroxyprogesterone acetate) or chronic disease such as rheumatoid arthritis.

Alendronate is the only bisphosphonate that is licensed for the treatment of osteoporosis in men. The value of testosterone replacement has not been well established, especially in eugonadal men. Almost all men under 65 and premenopausal women with osteoporosis probably warrant a referral to exclude a secondary cause. Screening blood tests would include a 9-am testosterone level, thyroid function tests (TFTs), routine biochemistry (including LFTs and calcium) and possibly endomysial antibodies for coeliac disease.

Lifestyle measures

- Increase dietary calcium to 1000 mg per day; 1 pint of milk taken with 1 pot of yoghurt (125 g) or 60 g of cheese will provide 1000 mg of calcium. Vitamin D is found in margarine and oily fish.

- Stop smoking.

- Reduce alcohol consumption if greater than the recommended limits.

- Exercise, eg walking, climbing stairs, dancing. Head-lifts are good for increasing back muscle strength: the patient should lie down on their front, with their hands folded under their forehead. They then lift their forehead off their hands. A rolled towel placed under the abdomen can help to reduce back discomfort. Eventually, the patient should aim to lie on their front, with their arms by the sides of their body, palms facing downwards. They should then raise their back, head and shoulders off the floor, keeping their hips and legs still. A useful leaflet is 'Exercise and Osteoporosis', published by the National Osteoporosis Society.

HOW OFTEN SHOULD DEXA SCANNING BE DONE?

Repeat DEXA scans should only be performed if doing so will influence treatment; there may not be any point in repeating a scan on someone who is already on alendronate or risedronate in combination with calcium/vitamin D supplements, especially if they have had no subsequent fractures. Patients with osteopenia who are not being treated with bisphosphonates may need to have a DEXA scan approximately every 3 years.

FALLS

It should be possible for most people to get up from a chair without using their arms, and then walk several paces without becoming unsteady (the 'get up and go' test). If they are unable to do this, they may be at increased risk of falling. In this case, their medication, BP (including postural drop), balance, osteoporosis risk, cognition, vision and hearing should be assessed, as well as any other treatable co-morbidities. Patients with multiple chronic diseases and those on several drugs are at increased risk of falls.

NICE recommends that elderly patients should be routinely asked about falls, and assessed as above if they have fallen. Patients should receive a 'multifactorial assessment', usually in a specialist falls clinic. Useful interventions include physiotherapy to improve strength and balance and occupational therapy to see whether any adjustments can be made at home.

OSTEOMALACIA

Osteomalacia most often presents in Asian women living in the UK and in the elderly. The most common cause is vitamin D deficiency, secondary to an inadequate diet, lack of sunlight or malabsorption. Asians and Africans need more sunlight than Caucasians to produce the same quantities of vitamin D. Osteomalacia may present with bony pains (as opposed to joint pains) and proximal muscle weakness; the pain is usually symmetrical, starting in the lower back and spreading to the pelvis, upper legs and ribs. Calcium levels may be slightly low and alkaline phosphatase (ALP) can be raised (although this is not always so). Vitamin D levels can be approximated by measuring 25-hydroxycholecalciferol. Symptoms usually resolve after 3 months of treatment with oral calcium (1 g per day) and vitamin D (800 units, equivalent to 20 μg per day). Patients with malabsorption or anorexia nervosa will need intramuscular vitamin D. If a patient has osteomalacia in addition to osteoporosis, the former should be corrected first, before initiating treatment with a bisphosphonate.

Vitamin D defieciency is more common than most doctors realise, especially in the elderly. The consequent muscle weakness can lead to falls and fractures. Treating all elderly, housebound people with 800 IU vitamin D daily (or 1000,000 IU every 4 months) may be effective in preventing falls and reducing mortality (*BMJ* 2003; 326: 469–72).

INTERPRETING AUTOANTIBODY RESULTS

Autoantibodies can either be specific to a certain organ, eg parietal cell autoantibodies in pernicious anaemia, or more general, eg antinuclear antibodies (ANA). The presence of ANA and rheumatoid factor can indicate rheumatological disease.

Autoantibody	Disease association
Antinuclear antibodies (ANA) (present in 0–2% of 'normal' people, more often in the elderly)	**SLE** (present in 99% of cases), **chronic active autoimmune hepatitis** (75%), **Sjögren's syndrome** (60–80%), **systemic sclerosis** (80%) and **RA** (32% of adults, 76% of cases of juvenile RA)
Rheumatoid factor (present in 5–10% of 'normal' people)	**RA** (70–80%), **Sjögren's** (almost 100%), **Felty's syndrome** (almost 100%), **systemic sclerosis** (30%), **SLE** (<40%)
Double-stranded DNA	**SLE**
Antiphospholipid antibody	**SLE** and **associated with thrombosis and miscarriage**
Ro/La (SS-A/SS-B)	**SLE with Sjögren's syndrome**
Scl-70 and anticentromere antibodies	**Scleroderma/CREST syndrome**
Jo-1	**Dermatomyositis/polymyositis**

Table 16.2: Autoantibodies and their associated diseases

ANTINUCLEAR ANTIBODIES

The term 'antinuclear antibodies' is an umbrella term. There are various different nuclear and cytoplasmic antigens, and the pattern of antinuclear antibodies varies according to the disease. For example, a speckled pattern of staining occurs in mixed connective tissue disease and staining that occurs in the nucleolus is found in scleroderma. Sometimes the antinuclear antibody is negative, but there are specific nuclear antibodies (eg to Ro) which have not been detected.

Double-stranded DNA (dsDNA) antibodies and extractable nuclear antigen (ENA) antibodies are often tested if the ANA is positive, or if a patient is very symptomatic but has a normal ANA result. The presence of antibodies against ENA would be strongly indicative of an underlying systemic autoimmune disease. There are certain antibodies to ENA that are specific for particular conditions, eg anti-La and anti-Ro antibodies occur in Sjögren's syndrome; anti-Sm antibodies occur in SLE; and Scl-70 antibodies may be found in scleroderma. High serum levels of dsDNA antibodies are very specific for SLE, although lower levels can be found in scleroderma and polymyositis.

In practice, if an ANA is positive in primary care, the patient should almost always be referred if they are symptomatic, and further testing will be done in the secondary care setting. Conversely, if a patient has suspicious symptoms, eg arthritis in conjunction with a rash, but their ANA is negative, they should still be referred.

CHAPTER 17
UROLOGY

CHAPTER 17
UROLOGY

FORESKIN PROBLEMS

Around 50% of 1-year-old boys have a non-retractile foreskin ('physiological phimosis'); if left alone, this reduces to 15% at 3 years and 1% at 16 years. Conditions affecting the foreskin include recurrent infections, ballooning and balanitis xerotica obliterans (BXO). BXO is also known as 'lichen sclerosus' and is the only absolute indication for circumcision. It is characterised by pallor, scarring and stenosis of the prepuce and is rare in boys under 5 years old.

Ballooning is most common between the ages of 2 and 4 years and generally resolves as the foreskin becomes more easily retractable. Until this happens it can be managed by advising gentle retraction of the foreskin during urination, so that the urethral meatus is apposed to the opening of the prepuce.

Balanoposthitis describes an acute pyogenic infection of the foreskin characterised by erythema, oedema and a purulent discharge. It is best managed with topical antibiotics and is very different from what is commonly referred to as 'balanitis', ie erythema with or without oedema with **no** purulent discharge. A degree of balanitis occurs naturally with the spontaneous lysis of preputial adhesions and often occurs in young boys who 'fiddle' with their foreskin. The parents can be reassured that this will generally settle if left alone. Topical steroid cream (eg betamethasone (Betnovate®) 0.05% bd for 1–2 months) has been shown to accelerate the lysis of preputial adhesions, thereby speeding up the process of retractibility, and can be tried with persisting prepuce problems. Should all this fail, then referral for a urological opinion is reasonable.

Paraphimosis is when the foreskin has been retracted for a period and cannot be replaced, due to the venous engorgement and oedema that are commonly present. It is often acutely painful and patients are usually very anxious about what you are going to do to them. Management in the first instance consists of gently squeezing the glans for a period of 5–10 minutes to reduce the oedema. In most cases the foreskin can then be replaced. If this fails, patients should be referred to the on-call urology team; a dorsal slit or circumcision may be required.

URINARY TRACT INFECTION

Urinary tract infections (UTIs) in men are unusual and there is a reasonably high chance of underlying pathology. Confirmed UTIs should therefore be referred for a urological opinion. Similarly, any child with a UTI should be referred to a paediatrician.

In contrast, UTIs are common in both pre- and postmenopausal women and are often recurrent. Initial assessment should include:

- History, for example of diabetes mellitus or triggering factors such as sexual intercourse.

- Examination: a palpable bladder may be demonstrated and atrophic vaginitis should be excluded in postmenopausal women.

- Urinalysis and mid-stream urine (MSU).

INTERPRETING THE MSU RESULT

Leucocytes on microscopy or on dipstick analysis frequently signify infection, and, conversely, infection is rare in the absence of pyuria. It is worth noting that urine culture is not 100% sensitive, so a negative MSU does not always exclude infection; this may explain some cases of the so-called 'urethral syndrome', in which women with sterile urine on MSU complain of dysuria.

'Mixed growth' is a common finding and, in the absence of pyuria, is unlikely to be significant.

Further investigations in persistent cases include ultrasound scan of the renal tract, abdominal radiography and flexible cystoscopy.

Management includes general lifestyle advice:

- Ensure fluid intake >2 l/day

- Cotton underwear

- Void after intercourse (generally within 1 hour)

- Avoid adding products to bathwater

- Cranberry juice/capsules - several studies have shown that cranberry juice helps to reduce recurrent UTIs (*Cochrane Database Systematic Review* 2004; (1): CD001321); although the doses vary between studies, generally 200 ml tds is reasonable

- Probiotic supplements – may have a role in altering perineal microflora but not proved in a randomised controlled trial yet.

Acute UTIs should be treated according to the MSU sensitivities (although resistance demonstrated in a lab setting does not always apply in vivo). Generally, a 3-day course of antibiotics is sufficient for uncomplicated UTI in women, but longer courses are usually needed if there is evidence of pyelonephritis or if the patient is pregnant. Men and children may also need longer courses.

Usual first-line options are trimethoprim or nitrofurantoin. The latter is also available as a twice-daily sustained-release preparation. Cefalexin should usually be reserved for resistant infection.

OPTIONS FOR PROPHYLAXIS OF RECURRENT UTI

Medical treatments should only be used if lifestyle measures fail:

- Topical oestrogen cream may be helpful in patients with atrophic vaginitis, although recent studies have shown that it may also be of use in premenopausal women.

- Antibiotic prophylaxis (eg trimethoprim 100 mg nocte, nitrofurantoin 50–100 mg od or ciprofloxacin 125 mg od) should be considered when conservative measures have failed.

- For UTIs associated with sexual intercourse, a single dose of antibiotic taken postcoitally may be of benefit (eg trimethoprim 200 mg or nitrofurantoin 100 mg).

Recurrent or persistent UTIs should be referred for further urological investigation. There is no good evidence to define exactly what is meant by recurrent infection, but proved infection more than three times per year probably justifies referral to exclude underlying disease such as a bladder stone or bladder diverticular disease.

HAEMATURIA

Haematuria may be microscopic or macroscopic: either of these may be painful or painless.

Painless macroscopic haematuria and persistent microscopic haematuria (on more than one occasion) are indications for referral to Urology Outpatients as part of the 2-week cancer initiative. Overall, a pathological cause (including UTI) will be found in up to 40% of patients. Generally, fewer than 1% of patients with persistent microscopic haematuria will be found to have a urothelial malignancy. Useful initial investigations include:

- MSU
- Urine cytology
- Kidney-ureter-bladder (KUB) ultrasound
- Abdominal (KUB) radiography.

Painful macroscopic haematuria should be treated in the first instance with antibiotics while awaiting MSU results. Should the MSU prove negative, a urological referral for further investigation is required.

Further investigation in secondary care will usually involve a flexible cystoscopy; this is done as a day case procedure under local anaesthetic.

Heavy haematuria with clots and very painful haematuria (including clot retention) should be referred urgently to the on-call team.

MANAGEMENT OF LOWER URINARY TRACT SYMPTOMS (LUTS)

LUTS secondary to benign prostatic hypertrophy are a common complaint amongst men over the age of 40. Initial assessment almost invariably takes place in the primary care setting and should involve the following:

- History, including IPSS (International Prostate Symptom Score; see http://tinyurl.com/6lats). A score on the IPSS of >19 indicates that the symptoms are severe. Try to differentiate between obstructive ('voiding' symptoms) and irritative ('storage' symptoms) problems. Voiding symptoms include poor stream, hesitancy and terminal dribble. Storage symptoms include increased frequency, nocturia, urgency and incontinence.

- Examination should include palpation for a bladder and digital rectal examination (DRE).

- Urinalysis ± MSU.

- Prostate-specific antigen (PSA), always after counselling, and when a positive result would change management. PSA is also a good measure of the size of the gland.

The following warrant urgent urological referral:

- Macroscopic haematuria

- Acute retention of urine

- Chronic retention of urine in the context of renal failure

- Suspicious DRE or abnormally raised PSA.

UTIs should be treated appropriately before re-assessment; UTIs will raise PSA levels and cause false-positive results.

Patients with nocturia should be assessed for nocturnal polyuria (suspect if nocturia more than three times a night) by means of a voiding diary. This will demonstrate if large volumes of urine are being passed at night, in which case reduction in evening/night-time drinking should be advised. If the voiding diary indicates small volumes, then an underlying bladder or prostate problem is more likely.

Treatment begins with lifestyle advice, eg cutting out night-time drinks and reducing caffeine intake. Should this fail, then alpha-blockers offer the potential for rapid improvement in symptoms; they relax the muscle in the prostate/bladder neck and are effective within hours.

Patients with an enlarged prostate (more than 30 ml) or raised PSA (more than 1.4 ng/ml) are at risk of their symptoms worsening and ultimately of acute retention. These men may benefit from combination therapy with alpha-blockers and 5-alpha-reductase inhibitors (which shrink the prostate over a matter of months) as well as lifestyle changes.

Five-alpha-reductase inhibitors such as finasteride reduce PSA levels by approximately 50%. Therefore, to get an accurate reading, the PSA result obtained should be doubled in these patients.

Herbal alternatives include saw palmetto, the African plum, the nettle and pumpkin seeds; all have been shown to be effective (*Journal of Urology* 2000; **163**: 1408-1412).

If medical management fails or is not tolerated, then a referral for urological opinion with regards to surgery is appropriate. In general, surgery is more effective for men with predominantly obstructive symptoms and may actually worsen irritative symptoms.

Indications for surgery include:

- Failure of medical treatment
- Moderate or severe symptoms (IPSS >7)
- Refractory urinary retention
- Large post-void residual urine volumes (>100 ml)
- Recurrent UTIs
- Recurrent persistent gross haematuria
- Bladder calculi
- Renal failure secondary to outflow obstruction.

Although standard electrosurgical transurethral resection of the prostate remains the gold standard, several new modalities, including holmium laser, green light laser, radiofrequency ablation and microwave treatment are available in some centres. The effectiveness of these new therapies in the long term has yet to be proved.

PSA TESTING AND INTERPRETING THE RESULTS

PSA as a blood test is used in prostate cancer for two main purposes: as a marker for disease progression following diagnosis, and (in combination with a digital rectal examination) as a screening tool for prostate cancer. PSA is **prostate**-specific, but not **cancer**-specific and generally two-thirds of patients with a raised PSA do not have prostate cancer. Other causes of a raised PSA include UTIs, prostatitis, retention of urine, benign prostatic hyperplasia (BPH), age, ejaculation (within 24 hours), vigorous exercise, and surgery or instrumentation to the prostate.

A raised PSA implies that further investigation (in the form of prostatic biopsy samples) is required to rule out or confirm the diagnosis of prostate cancer. With this in mind, PSA testing should never be performed without prior counselling.

There is at present no national screening programme for prostate cancer in this country. However, men should be offered the PSA test if they request it and following counselling. Men who may be suitable for screening in this manner are the over 50s and those over 45 who are either Afro-Caribbean or who have a strong family history. PSA testing is also part of the assessment of LUTS. Patients with a borderline PSA result (ie less than 10 ng/ml) and a normal digital rectal examination should generally have a repeat PSA carried out 4–6 weeks later before undergoing biopsy sampling.

PSA testing is **not** suitable for asymptomatic men who have less than a 10-year life expectancy.

Previously, the upper limit of normal for a PSA was considered to be 4.0 ng/ml. However, this missed a significant number of cancers in younger men. The normal ranges for PSA have now been stratified according to age and this has helped to reduce unnecessary biopsies (Table 17.1).

Age (years)	Age-adjusted PSA (ng/l)*
40–49	<2.5
50–59	<3.5
60–69	<4.5
70–79	<6.5

*These are subject to local variations

Table 17.1: Age-adjusted PSA

If the ratio of free to total PSA is <20%, prostate cancer is more likely. Conversely, the higher the ratio, the higher the chance of benign disease.

INCONTINENCE MANAGEMENT IN PRIMARY CARE

Incontinence may be divided into the following categories:

1 Incontinence associated with physical activity (stress incontinence)

2 Incontinence associated with urgency and/or frequency (urge incontinence)

3 A mixed picture of stress and urge incontinence

4 Overflow incontinence

5 Incontinence with a complex history (eg surgery, haematuria, pain, recurrent infections).

The latter two types often require specialist management but the first three may be managed (at least initially) in the primary care setting, especially with the support of community-based continence advisors.

Initial assessment should involve:

- History: voiding diaries are a useful adjunct (ie how frequently the patient urinates, and how long they spend urinating each time).

- Physical examination: the bladder should be palpated and the patient asked to cough, in order to demonstrate stress incontinence.

- Urinalysis ± MSU.

Further assessment with an ultrasound of the kidneys and bladder is often useful and allows the residual volume to be calculated. Patients with significant residual volumes (more than 10% of their bladder capacity, usually >100 ml) require specialist referral to determine the cause. The underlying aetiology is generally obstruction (eg from a large prostate or a urethral stricture) or bladder failure, or a combination of these.

Uncomplicated stress incontinence should initially be managed with lifestyle changes, pelvic floor exercises and bladder retraining (see Chapter 7, Gynaecology). Further therapies include specialised physical equipment such as vaginal cones and medical treatment with duloxetine. Surgery is indicated if these measures fail.

Urge incontinence is initially managed with lifestyle modifications, bladder retraining and antimuscarinics. If a mixed picture exists, then the most bothersome aspect should be treated first.

Lifestyle changes include: cessation of smoking, reduction in caffeine and alcohol intake, avoidance of fizzy drinks, and weight loss in the obese.

LONG-TERM URETHRAL CATHETERS

Long-term catheters are most commonly used in two groups of patients:

1 The elderly with incontinence, bladder outflow obstruction or bladder failure

2 Patients with spinal injuries or other neurological conditions that affect bladder function.

Common problems with long-term urinary catheters include:

- Discomfort/pain

- Spasm

- Bypassing

- Blockage

- Discharge

- Urinary tract infection.

One of these problems may occur in isolation or there may be several problems that co-exist.

- Discomfort/pain can be caused by bladder spasm, catheter blockage or infection. Treatment for spasm includes anticholinergics, reducing the volume of the balloon and avoiding caffeinated drinks.

- Blocked catheters should generally be replaced rather than flushed, and the underlying cause of the blockage addressed. This can usually be achieved by increasing fluid intake to at least 2 l/day and treating any underlying infection. Cranberry juice is particularly useful as it increases fluid intake and also has antibacterial properties. However, it should not be used in patients on warfarin. Bladder washouts can be helpful in those who cannot drink enough; they can help to reduce encrustation and recurrent blockage. Saline washouts are commonly used, or more specialised acidic solutions if the urine is alkaline (eg mandelic acid for *Proteus* and *Pseudomonas* infections). High oral doses of vitamin C will also acidify the urine and help prevent encrustation. A larger-diameter catheter can also help to reduce recurrent blockage but may cause increased pain and discharge.

- Catheter blockage can also be caused by kinking of the catheter itself, constipation and bladder spasms.

- Discharge from the urethra is common. In the uncatheterised urethra, paraurethral gland secretions are washed out with micturition. Catheters prevent this from happening and so the secretions present as a discharge around the edge of the catheter; this is normal. If the paraurethral glands become blocked, urethritis can occur, which is associated with a more profuse, often offensive-smelling, discharge. Problems with this can be reduced by using a smaller diameter catheter, ie 12 F. Smaller catheters are also more comfortable and can help to reduce pain and spasm.

Urinary infection is commonly diagnosed, but rarely needs treatment; asymptomatic bacteriuria is considered normal in catheterised patients. However, signs of sepsis should be treated with antibiotics and the catheter replaced to remove the existing biofilm.

Most long-term catheters can last up to 3 months. However, they may require changing more frequently and this varies from patient to patient.

ERECTILE DYSFUNCTION (ED)

ED is defined as the persistent (6 months) inability to achieve and maintain an erection sufficient for satisfactory sexual performance. Most men who suffer from this problem will initially present to a primary care physician.

Initial assessment should include:

- Medical history, including co-morbidities that may contribute to ED and drugs that cause it. This will also help the patient converse about the sexual history.

- Sexual history, preferably with a partner present. Importantly, patients should be asked about libido and spontaneous/nocturnal erections. If these are lacking, there may be a hormonal cause and a hormone profile should be taken (see below).

- Physical examination: this should include a digital rectal examination in those over the age of 50 years; prostate cancer that has extended beyond the capsule can lead to ED and haemospermia.

- Investigations include blood tests for diabetes mellitus, hormone levels (if low libido) and possibly PSA and lipids.

Hormone levels should be taken at 9 am as this is when testosterone peaks. Tests should include testosterone, follicle-stimulating hormone (FSH) and luteinising hormone (LH). A low testosterone with high levels of FSH and LH indicates primary gonadal failure and can be treated with testosterone replacement (available as gel, injections, or patches), except in patients with prostate cancer, for whom testosterone supplementation is contraindicated. Low testosterone levels with a normal or low FSH and LH are more consistent with hypothalamic or pituitary disease and this warrants referral to an endocrinologist.

The development of phosphodiesterase (PDE) inhibitors (eg tadalafil, sildenafil and vardenafil) has revolutionised the treatment of ED in recent years and these are now used as first-line treatment alongside psychosexual counselling, vacuum devices and sublingual apomorphine. They are contraindicated in patients who take nitrate medication, due to the profound hypotension that ensues when these drugs are taken concomitantly. PDE inhibitors are available on the NHS to men with the following conditions:

- Prostate or radical pelvic surgery (**not** including transurethral resection of the prostate (TURP))

- Prostate cancer

- Diabetes mellitus

- Severe pelvic or spinal cord injury

- Renal failure

- Multiple sclerosis

- Spina bifida

- Parkinson's disease

- Poliomyelitis

- Single gene neurological disease.

Men who were diagnosed and treated on the NHS before 1998 are also entitled to NHS prescriptions, as are men who are 'severely distressed' by the condition (although this is difficult to define unambiguously and should usually be diagnosed by a psychiatrist). All men can be prescribed PDE inhibitors on a private prescription basis. Apomorphine may be a useful medical alternative in patients taking nitrate medication.

If one particular PDE inhibitor is not effective, then it is worth trying another.

Second-line treatments include intracavernosal and intraurethral therapies. These can be very effective, but patients (or their partners) need to be manually dextrous in order to administer them. Third-line treatments consist of prosthetic surgery.

SCROTAL PAIN

Scrotal pain may be acute (lasting a few hours or more) or chronic (generally more than 6 months).

Any acute pain arising in the scrotum must be assumed to be testicular torsion until proved otherwise. Testicular torsion, epididymitis and torsion of a testicular appendage make up 85–90% of all cases of acute scrotal pain. These may be indistinguishable clinically and therefore immediate referral is essential to avoid potential loss of the testis.

Chronic scrotal pain is a frequent complaint and is a common outpatient referral. It may be constant, intermittent, unilateral or bilateral.

Clinical examination is important to localise the pain within the scrotum (ie testis or surrounding structures) and this includes groin examination to exclude hernias. Urinalysis should be performed and an MSU sent. Ultrasonography is often helpful to identify the cause and is mandatory for any male at risk from testicular cancer, as up to a third of cancer cases originally present with testicular ache/pain.

Intrascrotal lesions that may account for testicular pain include:

- **Torsion of the testis:** the testis may be high-riding with a horizontal lie, and there may also be some scrotal erythema. However, the only way to exclude this diagnosis for certain is to explore the scrotum surgically.

- **Torsion of a testicular appendage:** this is probably the commonest cause of testicular pain in children and adolescents. In children a black dot may be seen through the scrotal skin on the testis, although exploration is often required to make this diagnosis.

- **Infection:** epididymo-orchitis is a common cause of scrotal pain. In young, sexually active males it is most commonly caused by *Chlamydia* and should be treated with a 2-week course of doxycycline in the first instance. In older males, other organisms are more common, eg *Escherichia coli*. These can be treated with oral ciprofloxacin. As a rule of thumb, most cases should be treated first-line with ciprofloxacin and if *Chlamydia* infection cannot be excluded, doxycycline should be added. Recurrent infection may be due to the partner of the patient re-infecting them with *Chlamydia*. Generally, when *Chlamydia* is suspected, the patient should be referred to a Sexual Health Clinic, and if he tests positive his partner should be screened as well.

- **Tumour:** the testis is smooth and olive-shaped with the epididymis lying posteriorly. Any irregular lumps palpated on the body of the testis should be referred urgently; most urologists will see such cases in their next clinic.

- **Epididymal cysts:** on palpation, these are found to be separate from the body of the testis, and with experience, examination alone is sufficient to make the diagnosis. They can be managed conservatively unless they cause considerable pain, in which case referral for removal is indicated.

- **Varicocele:** this is a collection of dilated veins in the spermatic cord, which may present as chronic scrotal ache. Opinion is divided on whether all of these need surgery. The main risk of conservative management is a reduction in sperm count and testicular size over a long period. Generally, it is reasonable to treat large symptomatic varicoceles in younger men.

- **Hydrocele:** this is a collection of fluid in the tunica vaginalis and can be managed conservatively. They are not usually painful but problems tend to arise as they increase in size, and at this point referral for surgery is appropriate.

- **Postsurgical problems,** eg hernia repairs and granulomata after vasectomy.

- **Trauma:** This is mostly blunt trauma. Provided both testes can be fully palpated and the examiner is satisfied that there is no evidence of a ruptured testis, an outpatient ultrasound can be arranged and pain managed with simple analgesia. If the testes cannot be adequately palpated or if there is a large haematoma, then immediate referral is appropriate.

- Another important diagnosis is **intermittent torsion**, which when suspected should be referred urgently for orchidopexy.

Extragenital lesions causing referred pain to the scrotum include aortic aneurysm, urinary tract calculi, vertebral disease and constipation in children.

If investigations fail to yield a cause of the pain, then conservative management is employed in the first instance, ie oral analgesics, scrotal support, lifestyle changes (eg changing bicycle seats). Nerve blocks can be both therapeutic and diagnostic but ultimately surgical exploration may be necessary.

OTHER UROLOGICAL DIAGNOSES NOT TO BE MISSED

Many of the important areas in urology relevant to primary care have already been covered. Other important diagnoses include:

- **Renal colic.** This should be referred to hospital for investigations and management. An infected obstructed kidney presents with fever, rigors and loin pain. This is a life-threatening condition and should be referred immediately, as the kidney will require drainage with stenting or a nephrostomy.

- **Spinal cord compression.** Prostate cancer commonly metastasises to bone. Any patient with known prostate cancer who presents with severe back pain and neurological symptoms/signs should be referred immediately. They require an emergency MRI and treatment with dexamethasone prior to urgent radiotherapy.

- **Renal trauma.** This may be blunt or penetrating. All penetrating injuries require immediate referral. All children with blunt renal trauma should be referred. In adults, a history of blunt renal trauma with microscopic haematuria may be managed conservatively, as long as they do not have haemodynamic instability. Frank haematuria or any episode of haemodynamic instability should be referred immediately. An urgent CT scan will assess the degree of renal injury and direct management required.

- **Pelvi-ureteric junction (PUJ) obstruction.** The characteristic history of loin pain after drinking large volumes of fluid (Dietl's crisis) is not always present. Most commonly this diagnosis is made incidentally during investigations for other conditions or as part of antenatal ultrasound screening. A nuclear medicine scan will determine whether a pyeloplasty or nephrectomy should be performed.

CHAPTER 18
MISCELLANEOUS TOPICS

CHAPTER 18
MISCELLANEOUS TOPICS

SLEEP HYGIENE

Patients commonly come to their GP complaining of insomnia. Simple, non-medical strategies should always be tried first. These include:

- Ask the patient to reduce their consumption of alcohol and tobacco (especially around bedtime). Enquire about their use of over-the-counter (OTC) medication such as decongestants and of any illicit drugs.

- Avoid caffeine.

- Establish a regular time to wake up, regardless of the time spent asleep.

- Avoid daytime 'siestas'.

- Avoid large meals or large quantities of fluid around bedtime.

- Try to increase exercise, but ideally not within 3 hours of bedtime.

- Make sure the bedroom is not too hot or noisy.

- Try to get blackout lining for the curtains to ensure that the room is completely dark.

- Don't watch television just before bedtime.

- Try not to spend too much time in bed when not sleeping: this is in order to stop the patient associating being in bed with struggling against insomnia. The patient should be advised to go to bed only when they are actively feeling sleepy and get out of bed again if they have remained awake for more than 20 minutes. In this case, they should be encouraged to leave the bedroom and listen to some soothing music or read until they feel sleepy again. They should not, however, expose themselves to bright lights.

- Relaxation techniques can be helpful, eg visualising a relaxing, pleasant scene and learning to ignore intrusive thoughts. Physical relaxation can help to achieve mental relaxation, eg taking a hot bath or taking up yoga or meditation.

- Cognitive behavioural therapy can help patients who suffer from insomnia as a result of being stressed or anxious.

Most patients should respond to these measures, but the difficulty always lies in persuading people to change their lifestyles, as with so many other chronic conditions. There is no 'quick fix' and the dangers of benzodiazepine use should be emphasised (see Chapter 14, Psychiatry). NICE does not recommend the use of benzodiazepine receptor agonists such as zaleplon, zolpidem and zopiclone over traditional benzodiazepines. However, there may be less of an issue of tolerance with these newer drugs and they have less of a 'hangover' effect than other benzodiazepines.

Medication is always a last resort and should only be used for 2–3 weeks.

BENEFITS

DISABILITY LIVING ALLOWANCE (DLA)

- There are two components: a care component and a mobility component. The care component is payable if there is a severe disability, such that the patient requires help with daily living activities. The mobility component is payable at the higher rate if the patient is unable/virtually unable to walk due to a physical problem. It is payable at the lower rate if the patient can walk but only under supervision.

- People aged up to 65 are potentially eligible (from birth for the care component or from age 3 years for the mobility component), as long as the disability has been present for at least 3 months and is expected to continue for a further 6 months.

- The care component is worth between £15.15 and £58.50 per week, depending on the level of disability. The mobility component is worth between £15.15 and £41.05 per week.

- The GP is obliged to confirm the disability if requested to do so.

ATTENDANCE ALLOWANCE

- This is payable to patients over the age of 65 who have a severe mental or physical disability, such that they require assistance with daily activities.

- The disability must have been present for at least 6 months.

ALLOWANCES FOR THE TERMINALLY ILL

- The terminally ill are entitled to the DLA or Attendance Allowance, depending on their age. To expedite payments, form DS1500 should be filled in by the GP.

BLUE BADGE SCHEME

- Any patient over the age of 5 years with significant mobility problems can apply for parking concessions.

- The GP will usually be paid £20.50 by the relevant local authority for providing the necessary information.

- Successful applicants will be entitled to park free of charge on parking meters, in resident-only bays and will be able to use disabled bays.

INCAPACITY BENEFIT

- People aged between 16 and 65 (or 60 for women) are potentially eligible.

- It pays between £55.90 and £72.15 per week, depending on whether it is short- or long-term.

- To qualify, the patient must initially be able to demonstrate incapacity for their usual job, and subsequently incapacity for any work.

- The GP is obliged to provide the patient with a Med 3 if there is consensus about the incapacity.

- A Med 4 only needs to be issued once, when the Jobcentre Plus informs the GP that personal capability assessment has been applied.

SEVERE DISABLEMENT ALLOWANCE

- No new claims have been allowed since 2000; patients should now apply for Incapacity Benefit instead.

MOTHER/CHILD BENEFITS

STATUTORY MATERNITY PAY (SMP)

- Working women are entitled to up to 26 weeks of payment, commencing any time from 29 weeks' gestation; this is providing that they have worked for the same employer for at least 26 weeks by the end of the 25th week of pregnancy and that they earn >£79 per week on average.

- It is paid at 90% of the average weekly earnings for 6 weeks, and then at a standard rate of £102.80 per week (as long as the pay is >£114.20 per week; if not, SMP will continue at 90% of the weekly pay).

- The woman must have a Mat B1 form and inform her employer at least 4 weeks before she plans to stop work.

FREE PRESCRIPTIONS

- Women are entitled to free prescriptions while pregnant and for the first 12 months after birth. Children get free prescriptions until the age of 16.

- A form FW8 needs to be filled in and sent off to the health authority.

FREE DENTAL CARE

- Women are entitled to free dental care while pregnant and for the first 12 months after birth; the form can be collected from the dentist.

MATERNITY ALLOWANCE

- For self-employed women or working women who are not entitled to SMP (eg if they changed jobs during pregnancy); again, payable for 26 weeks.

- The maximum weekly rate is £102.80.

- The woman will need a completed Mat B1 and form MA1.

- Women not even entitled to the maternity allowance will be eligible for 8 weeks of Incapacity Benefit if they have paid National Insurance contributions in the past year.

SURE START MATERNITY GRANT

- Pregnant women or new parents who receive Jobseeker's Allowance, Income Support, Family Credit or Disability Working Allowance may be eligible to receive £500 for each baby (in order to purchase things for the child).

A QUICK GUIDE TO COMMONLY USED DRESSINGS

GRANUFLEX®

- Good for dry, granulating pressure sores and other dry wounds.
- Mepilex® is an alternative.

AQUACEL®

- Good for 'wet' wounds that are not infected, including pressure sores.
- Iodosorb® is an alternative.

KALTOSTAT®

- Used for fungating, malodorous wounds.
- CarboFLEX® is an alternative, particularly if the wound is discharging.

IODOFLEX®

- Contains antiseptic, good for necrotic, 'wet' areas.

INADINE®

- Simple dressing, good for acute wounds.
- Mepore® is an alternative.

INTRASITE® GEL + TEGADERM®

- Useful for dry necrotic wounds.

LYOFOAM®

- Good for overgranulating wounds.

LYMPHOEDEMA

Lymphoedema is often overlooked due to a general belief that there is no effective treatment for it. However, this is not the case: good skin care is essential and elastic compression hosiery can also be beneficial. Patients should be educated about the importance of treating skin infections early and about the technique of simple lymphatic drainage. The principle of manual lymphatic drainage (MLD) is to drain the lymph away from congested regions (especially useful for swellings affecting the face, trunk and genitalia) and can be used in conjunction with multi-layer bandaging and exercise. MLD is a specialised technique and should only be performed by a qualified therapist. Simple lymphatic drainage is a less complicated version of MLD and can be practised by the patient or their carer.

Recurrent cellulitis is a major problem in patients with lymphoedema and often causes systemic upset. Prevention is important and the patient should be treated promptly for any localised infection such as tinea pedis or dermatitis. If cellulitis does occur, antibiotics should be used early and patients should usually have a supply at home. A good first choice would be amoxicillin 500 mg tds for 2 weeks (or erythromycin 500 mg qds for 2 weeks in penicillin-allergic patients). If there is no improvement within 3 days, the antibiotic should be changed to clindamycin 300 mg bd. In the presence of severe systemic upset, the patient will need to be referred to hospital.

Patients who suffer from recurrent attacks of cellulitis justify prophylactic antibiotics; the drug of choice is penicillin V 500 mg od (or 500 mg bd if the patient weighs more than 75 kg or if they suffer from breakthrough attacks of cellulitis at a lower dose).

COMPRESSION STOCKINGS AND TUBIGRIP®

There are three grades of compression stocking, 1, 2 and 3, with 1 being the least compressive and 3 being the most. Doppler pressures need to be checked before prescribing class 2 or 3 stockings for a patient with risk factors for peripheral vascular disease. Class 1 stockings are often adequate for mild ankle swelling, whereas class 2 stockings are better at preventing recurrent venous ulcer formation. Class 3 stockings may be needed to treat lymphoedema or severe post-thrombotic venous insufficiency.

All classes of compression stocking come in above- and below-knee varieties. There is also a compression sock available (the Activa® ribbed sock), which might be more acceptable to male patients. Below-knee stockings are usually prescribed for ankle swelling, but for uncomfortable varicose veins thigh-length stockings might be more suitable.

Tubigrip® can be used as an alternative to compression stockings if the patient is unable to tolerate stockings or has difficulty in putting them on; although less effective, it is easier to use. If extra support is needed, the Tubigrip® can be worn as a double layer. A rough guide to sizes is as follows:

- **A**   Infant feet and arms
- **B**   Small hands and arms
- **C**   Medium arms, small ankles
- **D**   Large arms, medium ankles, small knees
- **E**   Large ankles, medium knees, small thighs
- **F**   Large knees, medium thighs
- **G**   Large thighs.

THERAPEUTIC DRUG LEVEL MONITORING

Drug	Timing of test	Frequency of test	Normal range
Digoxin	6–12 hours after last dose	Routine monitoring not necessary but may need to check, eg if new medication introduced or patient otherwise unwell	0.8–2 µg/l
Lithium	12 hours after last dose	Every 3 months once stable (with thyroid function tests (TFTs) every 6 months)	0.4–1.0 mmol/l
Phenytoin	Trough level (just before next dose)	For dosage adjustment	10–20 mg/l ($\equiv$ 40–80 µmol/l)

Other anti-epileptics do not have to be monitored routinely, unless the doctor wishes to check compliance or suspects toxicity.

FAMILIAL RISK OF BREAST CANCER (NICE 2004)

The question of whether to refer women with a family history of breast cancer is one that is frequently posed in general practice. NICE have recently issued guidance about which women should be referred.

For the purposes of assessing risk, a first-degree relative is defined as a parent, a child or a sibling. A second-degree relative is defined as a grandparent, a grandchild, an aunt or uncle, niece or nephew, or half-brother or half-sister.

The following women are at high risk of developing breast cancer (>30% lifetime risk) and should be referred:

- One first-degree female relative **and** one first- or second-degree female relative on the same side of the family diagnosed below an average age of 50 years

- Three or more first- or second-degree female relatives on the same side of the family diagnosed at any age

- One first-degree male relative diagnosed at any age

- One first-degree relative with bilateral breast cancer, where the primary was diagnosed before the age of 50 years

- One first- or second-degree relative with ovarian cancer at any age **and** one first- or second-degree female relative with breast cancer at any age.

The following women are at 'moderate' risk (defined as a lifetime risk of 17–30%) of breast cancer and should be referred to secondary care to discuss extra screening if they are aged between 40 and 49 years or if they are keen to have risk management advice:

- One first-degree female relative diagnosed below the age of 40 years

- One first-degree female relative **and** one second-degree female relative on the same side of the family diagnosed after an average age of 50 years

- One first-degree female relative with bilateral breast cancer, where the primary was diagnosed after the age of 50 years

- Two first-degree relatives on the same side of the family diagnosed after an average age of 50 years.

Women with only one relative diagnosed with breast cancer above the age of 40 years should be managed in primary care **unless** any of the following apply (in which case referral should be discussed with a specialist):

- There is a paternal history of breast cancer.

- There is Jewish ancestry; Jewish women are five to ten times more likely to be carriers of the BRCA1 or BRCA2 mutations than other women.

- There is a family history of unusual cancers (eg bilateral breast cancer, male breast cancer, ovarian cancer, sarcoma <45 years of age, glioma, multiple cancers at a young age).

USEFUL CONTACT INFORMATION

Action for Blind People: information, advice and grants for the blind (including help with employment issues)

Tel. 020 77328771

Age Concern: useful information on issues such as state benefits and care. Has local branches, which provide different services, such as meals on wheels, home visits, help with gardening, etc, according to local funding

Tel. 020 87657200

Helpline 0800 009966

www.ageconcern.org.uk

Al-Anon Family Groups: support for families and friends of alcoholics and ex-alcoholics, including a special service for teenagers affected by others' drinking.

Helpline (24-hour) 020 74030888

Alcohol Concern: national umbrella body for 500 local agencies tackling alcohol-related problems and providing support for families of alcoholics. It funds a helpline called the 'drink line' and can put patients in touch with a suitable local agency that will provide help with detox and general support for the patient and their family. The exact services available vary from region to region, according to available funding

Helpline (Drink Line) 0800 9178282 (open 9 am – 11 pm Mon–Fri & 6–11 pm Sat & Sun; has Urdu- and Gujarati-speaking volunteers)

www.alcoholconcern.org.uk

Alcoholics Anonymous

Helpline 020 78330022 or 0141 2262214 for Scotland

Alzheimer's Society: national society providing patient and family support as well as a good helpline. Website has patient information sheets and details of local support groups

Membership line 0845 3060868

Helpline 020 73060606

www.alzheimers.org.uk

Amarant Trust: provides information on all aspects of the menopause

Helpline 0901 6070312

Administration 01622 870041

www.amarantmenopausetrust.org.uk

Anxiety management 'No Panic': helpline, information leaflets and self-help groups for anxiety sufferers

Helpline 0808 8080545

Information line 0800 7831531

Arthritis Care: information for patients with arthritis

Helpline 020 73806555

www.arthritiscare.org.uk

Benefits Enquiry Line: information on sickness and disability benefits

Helpline 0800 882200

www.dwp.gov.uk

British Pregnancy Advisory Service: can offer advice about contraception and terminations

Tel. 08457 304030

www.bpas.org

Cancerline UK: for cancer sufferers and their families, provides useful information and support

www.cancerlineuk.net

Carers UK: information and support for unpaid carers

Helpline 0808 8087777

Tel. 020 74908818

www.carersonline.org.uk

Chartered Society of Physiotherapists: information on all aspects of physiotherapy, including a list of registered practitioners

Tel. 020 73066666

www.csp.org.uk

Coeliac Society of the UK: comprehensive dietary advice for sufferers. A list of local groups can be found on the website

www.coeliac.co.uk

Continence Foundation: advice for sufferers of urinary and faecal incontinence

Tel. 0207 4046875

Helpline 08453 450165

www.continence-foundation.org.uk

CRUSE: support for the bereaved and their carers

Daytime Helpline 0870 1671677

Evening Helpline 08457 585565 (Mon–Fri 5–9 pm, Sat & Sun 3–5 pm)

Depression Alliance: for sufferers and their families

Tel. 0845 1232320

www.depressionalliance.org

Diabetes UK: information about managing diabetes mellitus

Tel. 0845 1202960

www.diabetes.org.uk

Disabled Living Foundation: information for disabled and older people (including those with dementia) on equipment that might help to promote their independence

Helpline 0845 1309177

Tel. 020 72896111

www.dlf.org.uk

Domestic Violence Helpline: support and help for victims

Tel. 0845 7023468

Eating Disorders Association: help, support and advice for sufferers

Adult Helpline 0845 6341414

Youth Helpline 0845 6347650

www.edauk.com

ERIC: Enuresis Resource and Information Centre

Tel. 0117 9603060

www.eric.org.uk

Family Planning Association

Tel. 0845 3101334

www.fpa.org.uk

Foundations: can organise for disabled and older home-owners and private sector tenants on low incomes to have free home improvements, to enable them to stay in their own homes

Tel. 01457 891909

www.foundations.uk.com

H-E-A-R-T UK: for patients with heart disease

Tel. 01628 628638

www.heartuk.org.uk

Home-Start UK: volunteers offer practical support to parents with at least one child under the age of 5 who are experiencing difficulties

Tel. 0116 233 9955

Irritable Bowel Syndrome Network: information for patients

Tel. 0114 2623253

www.ibsnetwork.org.uk

Mental Health Medication: information for patients

Tel. 020 73597443

www.elfrida.com/publ.html

MIND: information for patients with mental illness

Tel. 0845 7660163

www.mind.org.uk

National Association for Colitis and Crohn's Diseas: information for patients

Tel. 01727 844296

www.nacc.org.uk

National Asthma Campaign: helpline staffed by specialist nurse, offering help for all aspects of asthma management

Helpline 08457 010203

Tel. 020 72262260

www.asthma.org.uk

National Childbirth Trust

Tel. 0870 4448707

www.nct-online.org

National Osteoporosis Society: useful source of information on the disease for the patient

Tel. 01761 471771

Helpline 0845 4500230

www.nos.org.uk

NHS Pregnancy Smoking Helpline: for help with quitting

Helpline 0800 1699169

www.givingupsmoking.co.uk

NHS Smoking Helpline

Helpline 0800 1690169

Pain Concern: for pain sufferers and those who care for them

Tel. 01620 822572

www.painconcern.org.uk

Parentline (and the National Stepfamily Association): offers help and advice to parents on all aspects of bringing up children and teenagers. Provides support for parents under stress

Tel. 01702 554782

Helpline 0808 8002222

Partially Sighted Society: support for patients with some residual vision

Tel. 01302 323132

Rapport: counselling for couples with young families

Tel. 029 20811733

Relate: relationship counselling for couples or individuals >16 years of age. Sex therapy for couples. Clients pay on a sliding scale

Tel. 01788 573241

www.relate.org.uk

Ricability: a charity that researches, publishes and provides information on products for older people, including guidance on a wide range of community alarms and easy-to-use electrical devices

Tel. 020 74272460

www.ricability.org.uk

Royal National Institute for the Blind (RNIB)

Tel. 020 73912223

www.rnib.org.uk

SANE: aims to increase public awareness about mental illness, to promote research and to provide emotional support for patients with mental illness and their families. The helpline is open until 2 am daily

Tel. 08457 678000

www.sane.org.uk

Stroke Association: for patients and healthcare professionals

Helpline 0845 3033100

www.stroke.org.uk

Turning Point: help for people with drug and alcohol misuse problems and mental health issues. Nationwide agency: local numbers listed on website

www.turning-point.co.uk

Women's Health Information

www.womens-health.co.uk

INDEX